\*\*\*

It is my pleasure to endorse this book "Moderation Is Key." I have had the joy of knowing Owen, felt her passion for wellbeing.

I believe Owen has been given the mandate to equip and to help everyone in this day of busy lifestyles to be educated in the realm of being healthy.

Through experience, Owen has learned these valuable tools to pass on. I for one will look forward to putting into practice her helpful insights.

—**Wendy J Preston**, Pastor, *Faith Alive Church, Aylesbury Buckinghamshire. U.K.*

# Reviews For:

## *Moderation is Key*

I have read parts of 'Moderation Is Key' and found it to be engaging. This practical and well-written book is targeted at anyone who has struggled with their weight and is generally unfit.

Written in simple language, it draws on the real-life experiences of the author.

In addition, I have witnessed the author use the ideas in her book to assist people to get a grip on their weight.

Another dimension to the book is that it has the potential to draw people who desire to find the Lord to Him, as they start to see the depths of His love... and care.

Happy reading!

—**Ituah Ighodalo,** Senior Pastor, *Trinity House.*

\*\*\*

Owen Jones' youthful figure today is a true testimony of the food and exercise lifestyle routines she espouses in her incredibly simple-to-follow book.

I can honestly say that other friends and I, have witnessed Owen's incredible transformation from a rather well-rounded 17-year-old to the svelte figure she presented as a 28-year-old bride —a figure she has maintained consistently since then, albeit an even fitter version of her younger self.

As good friends over the years, we often meet up for lunch and I have no hesitation in testifying that Owen can really 'pack it in' but does so with a difference. Often making healthy choices, which she savors. She will sometimes treat herself to a dessert...she does not believe in deprivation.

Owen is very disciplined with her eating times, and will usually not eat after 7 pm. She has truly been an inspiration to us all.

**—Doreen Lambo**.

\*\*\*

In 2012, I lost over 50lbs, after years of believing it was impossible. This was the first time that I included The Lord in my weight loss goal. It was the most successful. Fast forward to 2018...I found myself struggling with weight gain.

Owen had been through significant weight loss and, more importantly, had kept it off for years. We spoke and I felt empowered and connected to God. A few months later, I was on course for achieving my goal. I praise God. I know that He used Owen as a key facilitator. Her coaching was so on point, encouraging. She just gets it!

**—Charis Ogbonna**.

\*\*\*

In the 25+ years that I have known Owen, she has been disciplined. She eats well daily (usually no later than 7 pm), and exercises, too. She has not only served herself well but has become an example of what happens when we are consistent and disciplined.

**—Tele Ogunfunmi**.

# Moderation is Key

## A Good Balance for a Healthy Lifestyle

Oghomwen (Owen) Jones

Published by KHARIS PUBLISHING, imprint of KHARIS
MEDIA LLC.

Copyright © 2021 Oghomwen (Owen) Jones

ISBN-13: 978-1-63746-026-9
ISBN-10: 1-63746-026-0

Library of Congress Control Number: 2021932923

Cover image by: Nina Grossfurtner

All KHARIS PUBLISHING products are available at special quantity
discounts for bulk purchase for sales promotions, premiums, fund-
raising, and educational needs. For details, contact:

Kharis Media LLC
Tel: 1-479-599-8657
support@kharispublishing.com
www.kharispublishing.com

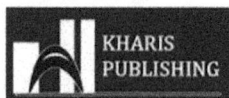

KHARIS
PUBLISHING

*This book is dedicated to God, The Captain of my destiny, who lit the fire within me that propelled me to share something about which I am so passionate: His love, a desire to fulfil His perfect Will, and His purpose for my life in conjunction with the pursuit of a healthylifestyle.*

*The photos included in the book are dedicated to my dear husband, John A. Jones, who passed away in 2017. I was very averse to letting them be seen. He often threatened to put them on the web. Now, with a change of heart, I have them in a book for the world to see.*

# TABLE OF CONTENTS

# Foreword

I was quite honored to be given the privilege to write the Foreword for *Moderation Is Key*. As you read this book, you will look at food differently.

I have been a nutrition consultant for seventeen years and enjoy watching the health of others improve and transform. We are all on different stages of our journey, some with more health challenges than others. We are all unique and different. No matter what phase or stage of life you are in, there is certainly something to take home from this book.

I was delighted and tickled reading *Moderation Is Key* from the other side of the table. It highlighted the very important aspects in which I counsel and encourage clients: listening to their body, staying connected, and being mindful.

Mrs. Jones, the author, gives her own experiences, and shares her opinions and thoughts. She has also uniquely and brilliantly intertwined Bible teachings and stories, relating them to many chapters. This I found to be very interesting.

*Moderation Is Key* allows the layman to understand the foundation of nutrition and its evolution from fad diets, metabolism, sugars, adverse reactions, and lifestyle. In my practice, we tie many of these premises to the foundation of disease and the journey of how to reverse it.

I certainly recommend this easy-to-read and practical book for those looking for a lifestyle change.

**—Sherese Ijewere.**

**Clinical Nutrition Consultant.**

# Acknowledgements

First and foremost, thank You Lord! Also, I thank my siblings. I am grateful to my sister, Itohan, for helping me see that it was all in me. She encouraged me to pray. I did--and watched this book unfold with her continued support. I thank my brother, Osahon, who also encouraged and shared interesting and informative podcasts and articles with me.

Thank you to my parents and my Pastor, Mr. Ituah Ighodalo, of Trinity House for their encouragement.

I acknowledge some of my friends for encouraging me and kindly sharing videos and articles. Tidbits from these references have been included in this book.

A big thank you to my dear friend Doreen Lambo and Pastor Tony Onyemaka of Trinity House, London. You both took the time and care to read the entire earlier book draft. Doreen, your constructive comments were very much appreciated. Pastor Tony, you were tremendously supportive. A big thank you to Mr. Samuel O. Towe who helped to format the book for publication.

Last, but not least, a big thank you to Yemisi Famuyide of Trinity House Lagos, who very kindly assisted me on social media. You patiently and kindly held my hand as I navigated this unfamiliar medium, during prepublication promotion.

# Chapter 1

# A Healthy Lifestyle

To enjoy a healthy lifestyle, we will ultimately have to engage our body, mind, and spirit in the process. The most important of these is our spiritual health. Without it, we will continually struggle with attaining our optimum physical health and spiritual growth.[1] In this book, I will dwell primarily on the importance of a body that is well cared for in our pursuit of a healthy lifestyle.

The health and wellness of our bodies are very closely related to what we eat and how we exercise. Our attitude towards these aspects of our lives will determine whether our lifestyle is healthy or not. Achieving such a lifestyle will involve engaging our minds, thinking[2] about what we put in our mouths, how we work out, how we rest, deal with stress and tackle other aspects of our lives. When we eat intentionally and endeavor to keep fit, we take huge steps towards improving our health and general well-being.

My primary aim in this book is to help you develop a healthy lifestyle, which will result in you feeling and looking your best. I want to help you step away from old, unhealthy habits and show you how to develop a new way of living. I will walk you through a way that will ensure that you take hold of the healthy life you truly want, and one you have likely dreamed about. Nobody--and I mean nobody--wants to be saddled with a tired, unfit, overweight, and sick body. There is a spring in our steps and a joyful approach to life when our bodies are functioning at their optimum. Trust me, I know what I am talking about. I was once overweight, and I want to share my experience with you. So please stay with me, and I promise you won't regret it.

It is important that we know from the onset that God loves us all. He wants us to live wholesome, healthy lives. The reason for this will become clearer as we continue to read. As Christians, our bodies are not our own. They are the temple of the Holy Ghost.

### 1 Corinthians 3:16 NIV
*Don't you know that you yourselves are God's temple and that God's Spirit dwells in your midst?*

### 1 Corinthians 6:19-20 GNT
*Don't you know that your body is the temple of the Holy Spirit, who lives in you and who was given to you by God? You do not belong to yourselves but to God; He bought you for a price. So use your bodies for God's glory.*

Some of us understand that God made our bodies, but perhaps we have never thought that they were made for Him. When we pursue excellence in every area of our lives, including our health, we honor God. We must stop making excuses about looking after our bodies.[3] When we are physically unhealthy, it is impossible to reach our full potential and fulfil the purpose God has for our lives. We really do not stand a chance or, at best, severely limit ourselves from doing so.[4]

You may be wondering, what is God's purpose for my life anyway? Ultimately, it is to glorify Him. How do you achieve this goal? One way is by living a healthy lifestyle. This will empower you to achieve God's unique purpose for your life. When you do this, you glorify God. Jesus glorified God by fulfilling all that His Father intended Him to.

### John 17:4 KJV
*I have glorified thee on the earth: I have finished the work which thou gavest me to do.*

You may be thinking, "What is God's purpose for me and how do I fulfil this in my life?" Let me say, emphatically, that we do not have any part in creating our purpose. Our Heavenly Father already has it all figured out. Just as our fingerprints are different, His planned role for each of us is unique. He has us all marked for a set role. We can begin by asking the Holy Spirit to help us seek and discover His lovingly thought out and unique plan and be prepared to walk in it.[5] God expects us to fulfil what He has called us to do--our purpose.

We need our bodies working at their optimum to fulfil God's purpose and enjoy our time here on earth. No body looks or feels as good as a well-fed and exercised one. Let's look at more scripture.

### Matthew 6:33 KJV
*But seek ye first the kingdom of God, and his righteousness; and all these things shall be added unto you.*

Matthew 6:33 says we should seek God first and His right way of doing things. When we do things His way, involving God in all that we do including eating the right way, we will have success and achieve the best results. We set ourselves up to be healthy and so have a good chance to accomplish all He has planned for us.

To those of you who are not Christians, I want to say that, without question, looking after your body and being methodical about preparing what you eat does not apply to Christians only. It applies to everyone. We only reach our full potential when we are healthy. It is only an intentionally looked after body that functions well and makes it through the day without being lethargic. God has a plan and purpose for each of us. He, however, does not force it upon us, as He always gives us free will.

Good health is necessary for the following:[6]

- Clear thinking

- Mental focus

- Enthusiasm

- Motivation

- Perseverance

- A quick response in an emergency and in times of danger

We must be deliberate about looking after our bodies; otherwise, our health and wellness may slowly start to spiral downwards and even gradually and/or eventually slip away from us. We must not let our days get so busy with the demands of family life, work concerns, and messy relationships to the detriment of our well-being. This often leads to minimal or no attention being paid to the way we fuel our bodies.[7]

We should willfully pay attention to our health and wellness and conduct our lives in such a manner as to ensure that we achieve the fullness of the life that God has for us. God has a plan for all areas of our lives, including our health. Our bodies are the living, breathing, and actualized temple of God's Spirit.[8] This reality has implications for how we care for ourselves physically, spiritually, emotionally, and mentally.[9] We should do all we can to make sure that we are at an optimum in all areas of our lives. God wants us all to live full, active lives, accomplishing the things He put us here for. Small, incremental steps are the key to successfully transition from an unhealthy lifestyle to a healthy one. We do not have to think that we must undergo an instant and extreme makeover to achieve our goals. Trying to do that is often a guaranteed setup for failure. Small deliberate steps will suffice; they can make a big difference.[10] Discipline will determine how well we follow through with the small steps that are required to realign our overall health and wellness with God's best plan for us.[11]

We should aim to focus on minor improvements every day, every week, and every month. There really are no quick fixes...easy does it. Over time, small, cumulative, intentional steps will be the best way to achieve our goals. If we are willing to make small, deliberate changes now, we can live a healthier life rather than suffer from the predictable results of mindless living.[12] These changes will help us avoid so many of the problems associated with a poor diet, such as excess weight, lack of sleep, and stress, to name a few. Being intentional about how we eat and exercise today will help ensure that we live our best lives for all our tomorrows.[13]

I cannot overemphasize enough that the path to our healthy future begins with the decision to stop wrestling with mediocrity[14] and to begin to eat and exercise thoughtfully. When we change the way we look after our bodies, we are likely to see many positive changes which will typically include weight loss, increased energy levels, and better sleep.

Eating and exercising intentionally is entirely up to us. No one can change our lives[15] without our participation. Let us make the changes required to live a healthy life. It will arouse those around us to be curious about the positive changes in us and be eager to know our secret.[16] Our improved lifestyle is likely to encourage them to want to know what we have learned and make them keen to step up their game and join us on our journey.

We can do this. Let's get started...

# Chapter 2

# Popular/Fad Diets

Let us start with a discussion of food that is required for general well-being. Later, in Chapter 8, we will look at the role of exercise in attaining our optimal physical goals.

Many fad diets out there promise a quick fix and typically limit a group or multiple groups of foods. The question is: Do they work? I do not believe that most of these diets work in the long-term. In my opinion, moderation and balance are key. When we eat moderate amounts of healthy food, which do not have to be boring or repetitive, and exercise moderately, we are likely to maintain a healthy weight and lifestyle.

## What are Fad Diets?

These are usually reducing diets that enjoy temporary popularity. In the times we live in, they are driven along exponentially by social media, which often generates a heightened interest, followed with exaggerated zeal.[1]

There have been many diets which encourage a low carbohydrate intake, such as the Keto (Ketogenic) and Dukan diets. Other diets are the Mediterranean Diet and the DASH Diet. DASH is an acronym for Dietary Approaches to Stop Hypertension.

The Keto Diet is currently very popular but, in a recent study by CNN, it ranked very low for long-term sustainability and health. The Mediterranean and DASH diets tied at first place. Some of these diets can perhaps be used to jump start a weight loss program but must be quickly replaced with a more sustainable and healthy eating plan.

Allow me to explain by taking a quick look at some of the current, popular diets individually.

## The Keto Diet

The Keto Diet is currently very popular. It is high in fats, moderate in proteins, and very low in carbs. It essentially cuts one's carb intake to a bare minimum. This diet aims to put the body into "ketosis." When the body is in this state, it breaks down both ingested and stored body fat into ketones and uses it for energy.[2]

There is no doubt that the Keto Diet can cause one to lose weight quite quickly. There is enough evidence that proves this. Its efficacy lies in its ability to raise ketone levels in our body. Apparently, under normal conditions our brains' and bodies' fuel of choice is carbs. When carbs are eliminated or greatly reduced, our bodies break down fats for fuel. However, our brain cannot burn fat, so our body has to come up with an alternate source of energy: ketones. These are a by-product of fat burning. When ketone levels get high enough, the body immediately begins burning fat as the primary fuel source instead of carbs. This switch speeds up fat loss.[3]

As I have already stated, that the Keto Diet will cause weight loss is not in dispute. However, we should not only be concerned with losing weight but keeping it off, too. Otherwise, we can quite easily become yo-yo dieters. I am not convinced that many find this way of weight loss sustainable. My main concern is with the foods one must forgo in order for weight loss to be effective, virtually no carbs are allowed. This, for me, is a deal breaker or a rule that is way too difficult to follow, as I imagine it is for many people. It should not be the crux of any eating plan, to want for so many foods in order to lose weight. For many, it just is not sustainable to do without a certain group of foods long- term. It certainly does not teach us how to acquire healthy eating habits. As long as we live, we have to eat. We will do well to develop a healthy relationship with food.[4]

According to nutritionist Lisa Drayer, a CNN contributor, The Keto Diet may be a good quick fix or jump start for weight loss, but most people can hardly give up bread and pasta, or beans and fruits, let alone a wide array of carbs. We really should not have to.

We must learn to be intentional about what we eat, and be favorably disposed toward healthy food choices. We need to eat the foods that we enjoy, mostly healthy in moderation. This low-carbeating plan may be helpful in managing type 2 diabetes. However, if we are not diabetic, there is nothing wrong in eating a sensible portion of healthy carbs. These are discussed in Chapter 3. Remember--moderation is key.

**The Dukan Diet[5]**

This diet promises to redesign one's eating habits and permanently stabilize the participant's weight. It is a high protein, low fat, and low carb diet with a food plan based primarily on proteins and vegetables—100 selected foods in total. It does not guarantee extreme results in record time. However, it promises that if instructions are strictly followed, a realistic amount of weight can be lost and maintained long-term. There are four phases to this eating plan.

**The Attack Phase**

This phase kick-starts the diet with 68 high protein meals and leads to immediate and noticeable weight loss. This phase typically lasts for one to seven days, depending on how much weight is to be lost.

## The Cruise Phase

In this phase, the aim is to reach your "true weight." Thirty-two vegetables are added in this stage. The plan here is to alternate pure protein days and protein + vegetable days. The length of this phase is based on a schedule of three days for each pound to be lost. The duration of this phase typically lasts anywhere from one to twelve months.

## The Consolidation Phase

This phase concentrates on the prevention of rebounding by reintroducing foods given up in the attack phase. Proponents of this diet claim that, at this time, participants are at their most vulnerable with a tendency to quickly regain weight lost. This is avoided by gradually introducing previously "forbidden foods" in limited quantities. The aim here is to curb cravings and possible bingeing of foods that were given up in the attack phase. The consolidation phase also allows the introduction of up to two indulgent meals per week. This phase typically lasts for five days for every pound lost.

## The Stabilization Phase

This relates to the rest of the participant's life. By this phase, healthy eating habits should have been learned. To maintain this, proponents suggest three non-negotiable rules:

- 3 tablespoons of oat bran a day

- A 20-minute daily walk and the choice of stairs wherever possible

- A pure protein day on the same day every week

In my opinion, the Dukan Diet may be healthier than the Keto Diet, as it is a low-fat diet compared to the latter's high fat content. However, the drawback again is the deprivation of some food groups such as no carbs in the first phase and "protein only" days. This may result in a possible negative impact on bowel movements. I believe another drawback is the limitation to only 100 foods, 68 initially and 32 added later. Also having to eat oat bran every day in the fourth phase would get monotonous quickly. In addition, our bodies require different exercise routines. A 20-minute daily walk would soon become boring as well as have minimal or no effect whatsoever. We need to mix up our exercise. This is discussed further in Chapter 8.

Another major flaw with this diet is the "protein day" on a specific day. What if we are invited out to an event with extraordinary food choices on that day? It would be a shame to miss out on these because of a diet. This rule will probably be a major drawback that sets us up to fail. I personally do not do well with food restrictions, and I strongly believe this is the case for most people. I tend to have more control when I am not limited in my choices, when I can eat what I want and enjoy them in moderation. I suspect this applies to most people.

## The Whole-30 Diet[6]

This diet was designed to change the way people eat and watch how they feel in 30 days and beyond. It involves the removal of all potentially inflammatory foods and beverages. These include junk foods (processed foods and beverages), dairy, grains, legumes, alcohol, added sugar, and sweeteners. Processed foods are discussed later in this chapter and extensively in *Chapter 5*.

The first phase of this eating plan lasts for 30 days and includes three meals a day that are "clean," containing only "whole-30" diet approved ingredients. These are primarily non-processed meats, seafood, vegetables, and eggs.

The second phase involves reintroducing the "un-healthy" foods that were excluded in phase one over the next 10 days and beyond, one group at a time. The rationale of reintroducing one group at a time is to better ascertain the "culprit" food with any adverse effects. These could be skin breakouts, achy joints, and bloating. An example would be to not reintroduce and eat a slice of toast and cheese at the same time, so that if there are any adverse reactions, we know whether it is the cheese or the bread that is the culprit. The rest of the diet is kept as "whole-30 clean" as possible. The plan here is to evaluate the way our body feels and reacts as we reintroduce foods that were eliminated in the first phase (the first 30 days) of the diet. The next two days following the reintroduction of foods are followed by two more days of going back to the "clean" whole-30 diet. We then re-introduce another food group, return to the "clean" whole-30 diet for another 2 days, and so on.

The general idea is that if there is a food or drink that we know makes us less healthy and one that we will not miss, there is no reason to reintroduce it. We should only reintroduce those "less healthy" foods that we would miss, but only occasionally.

Proponents of this plan see it as a jump-start to weight loss and a healthier way of eating. After the 30 days, they are mindful that people will probably slip back into their old habits. They encourage people to continue eating like the Whole-30 diet. In other words, avoiding added sugars and other food additives in processed foods. They also believe that it is ok to indulge occasionally if the food is truly enjoyed and done mindfully. In addition, if there is any major backsliding, they suggest restarting the whole-30 plan. It could be for 30 days or less, say 14 or 7 days, or just long enough to get back on track.

**The Paleo Diet[7]**

This eating plan advocates eating natural, unprocessed foods; it was the diet of cave men. It consisted of the animals they hunted and killed and other crops gathered. These were essentially foods in their rawest or truest form, available in nature. Their physiques were lean, muscular, and athletic. Other names for the Paleo Diet are Hunter-Gatherer Diet, Caveman Diet and Stone Age Diet.

Advocates of the Paleo Diet believe our bodies were physiologically created to be able to properly digest and derive energy from the original foods our ancestors ate. They are not genetically matched to the diets that emerged with modern day farming practices. The aim of this eating plan is to return to a way of eating that is more aligned with our early human ancestors. The foods in this plan are primarily nuts, seeds, fruits, eggs, freely roaming grass-fed animals, wild game, fish, healthy oils, and vegetables. Typically, these foods are eaten with minimal processing and are free of processed sugars and other additives.

The Paleo Diet excludes foods that became common when farming emerged about 10,000 years ago. Farming greatly influenced what people ate and introduced foods such as dairy products, legumes, potatoes, and grains as additional staples in the human diet. The Paleo diet also limits highly processed foods, refined sugars, and salt. Proponents of this diet claim that this relatively late and rapid change in man's diet outpaced the body's ability to adapt. This mismatch is believed to be the main reason for the prevalence of obesity, diabetes, and heart disease today. This eating plan also emphasizes drinking lots of water and being physically active every day.

The Paleo Diet is not just suggested for weight loss but is recommended for anyone who wants to feel and function better. Proponents of this way of eating apparently enjoy many health benefits. These include:

- Improved blood sugar control

- Improvements in cardiovascular health

- Weight loss

- Better sleep

I enjoy eating legumes and some dairy so would find the Paleo eating plan difficult. Legumes are a good source of fiber, vitamins, and other nutrients. Dairy has historically been a good source of protein and calcium (see discussion in the next paragraph); therefore, I would find it difficult eliminating these foods from my diet. It is hard though to argue against eating natural, unprocessed foods. After all, processed foods are linked to obesity, heart related diseases and many other ailments (see Chapter 5). You will see in Chapter 4 that I am extremely careful with processed foods.

I will include, ever so briefly here, my recent findings on dairy products. I have been paying more attention to milk and the ongoing discussions about it. Some of the reasons why we should reconsider animal milk consumption include:[8]

- Dairy milk actually robs our bones of calcium. Acid is a by-product of animal proteins. Calcium is an excellent acid neutralizer. Our bodies end up using the calcium that the milk contains in addition to some from our own stores to mop up the acid. Yikes!

- Dairy milk and cheese may increase the risk of prostate cancer.

- Dairy products increase our cholesterol levels.

- Dairy products can increase the prevalence and severity of acne in some adolescents and adults.

- Many cheeses have so much salt added to them. Salt is discussed further in *Chapter 5*.

Studies suggest that milk consumption in adults does not provide any real benefits. It has been found to provide no protection for men and an increased risk of fractures in women. I am still digesting the discussions on milk, and I admit I am struggling, as I do enjoy cheese. I also enjoy Greek yogurt, and thankfully it provides, among other benefits, probiotics, which are good bacteria that may restore a healthy gut bacterial balance.

It is very interesting to note that many common food allergies/intolerances are caused by foods introduced by modern farming practices. There are many adverse food reactions associated with:[9]

- Dairy Products – such as milk, cheese

- Legumes - such as beans and peanuts

- Grains - such as wheat, oats, and barley

These are discussed further in *Chapter 9*.

## The Mediterranean Diet[10]

Mediterranean populations generally have a healthy relationship with food: they eat well and enjoy their food. They live lives free from empty calories, unrealistic diet promises, and a "say no to food" mentality. This typically involves one seemingly being on a "diet" when around others but eating erratically when alone. This can be quite a damper, especially if there are only two people at a meal.

The Mediterranean approach to food, somewhat describes my way of eating. I eat well and enjoy my food. I describe my typical meals in some depth in Chapter 4. Mediterranean cuisine includes vegetables, fruits, whole grains, legumes, nuts, seeds, potatoes, fish, seafood, poultry, bread (eaten plain or dipped in olive oil), rice, pasta, herbs, spices, and extra virgin olive oil. With breads and pastas, we should choose wholegrain varieties where possible. This diet is also low in meat, eggs, and dairy products. It avoids processed meats, highly processed foods, sugar-sweetened beverages, trans-fats, refined grains, and oils. (See the paragraph below where I give a few examples of processed foods). I give a substantive narrative of these foods in *Chapter 5*.

The Mediterranean Diet ingredients are easy to find in the grocery store and contain nutrients that are known to enhance longevity and have other health benefits that are backed by peer-reviewed, scientific studies. A moderate amount of alcohol (one glass per day) is permissible regularly.

**Processed Foods**

These include processed meats, like hot dogs, sausages, cold cuts, etc. Other highly processed foods including all diet foods, margarine, microwave popcorn, and other packaged foods that are manufactured in a factory. Some more examples are foods like pasta and white bread made from refined grains and refined wheat. Some of these like margarine and microwave popcorn, contain trans-fats. These foods are discussed more extensively in *Chapter 5*.

The foods in the Mediterranean Diet are rich in flavor, have healthy nutrients, and are low in saturated fats and cholesterol.

**The DASH Diet[11]**

DASH is the acronym for dietary approaches to stop hypertension. It is promoted by the US based National Heart, Lung, and Blood Institute as a way to prevent and control hypertension. It is a diet rich in vegetables, fruits, whole grains, and low-fat dairy foods. It also includes fish, poultry, nuts, antioxidant rich foods, and beans. The DASH Diet limits salt, sugar-sweetened foods and beverages, red meat, saturated fats, and cholesterol. In addition to its positive effect on blood pressure, it is designed to give people a well-balanced eating plan.

In my opinion, the Mediterranean and DASH Diets are sustainable and ideal eating plans. They are similar to the way I like to eat, as will be discussed in *Chapter 4*.

## My Additional Opinions About Fad Diets

I really wonder if people on these diets truly enjoy their food. God cares about us enough to want us to enjoy what we eat. I discuss this attribute of God in Chapter 3. I think fad dieters, for the most part, long for foods that are restricted in their eating plans. I certainly would. In the past when I tried restricting food groups, I found myself really craving those foods, often uncontrollably. When there are no restrictions in place, I do not experience such cravings. It is best to make nutritious food choices and eat what we enjoy from these healthy selections in moderation. We must stop relying on the empty promises made by the proponents of unrealistic fad diets.

In my opinion, the long-term sustainability of most fad diets is rife with pitfalls. These are the main ones:

## Boredom

As with any diet with so many restrictions on the types of foods eaten, it can get irksome as meals quickly become repetitive and boring. To stay committed to a healthy eating plan, it is easier when we have a wide selection of healthy foods that we can choose from and enjoy. As they say, variety is the spice of life. We should work hard at not boring our taste buds and let them enjoy a wide range of foods. Again, moderation is essential here.

When one gets bored with one's eating plan, it is very easy to put back all the weight that was lost, and then some. The main reason this happens is because, oftentimes, people get frustrated and binge or eat erratically for a period.

I recall noticing the sudden and tremendous amount of weight lost by a lady I see from time to time. I wasn't sure what she did to lose that much weight. I was alarmed and asked her. She was very vague, said she was exercising a lot and on a diet. She was rather coy about divulging which one. I was not at all surprised when, after a very short period, she grew bigger than she was before her sudden, tremendous weight loss.

She probably started to crave the very foods avoided to lose weight and started eating them again uncontrollably. This is often the case with losing weight too quickly, as with long sustained fad dieting that has heavy restrictions on carbs. This lady could also have been on a crash diet. (See the effects of crash dieting in *Chapter 7*). A moderate weight loss plan is easier to sustain. It cannot be overemphasized that moderation is key.

## A Change in Bowel Movements

With a high protein and reduced carbs diet, and therefore most likely insufficient fiber as prescribed by some fad diets, how does one maintain regular bowel movements?

The foods we eat play a significant role in whether we are constipated and with our bowel movements in general. The Keto Diet can be an appetite suppressant. This is so because the fats recommended in this diet can be quite satiating. This encourages weight loss, and not eating much also reduces the frequency of bowel movements.

In addition, the keto diet has a strong diuretic effect in its induction phase. The resulting increased urine output often leads to constipation. Another possible cause of constipation with the Keto Diet is an imbalanced gut flora due to a higher fat intake.[12]

Low-carb diets can also make it easy to neglect key nutrients like magnesium, calcium, and potassium found in some high-carb foods like beans, bananas, and oats. These foods are high in fiber, too. Other fiber-rich foods like whole grains, brown rice, wholewheat bread, and pasta are excluded or greatly minimized in low-carb diets. So are starchy fruits, which include raisins and plums. Starchy vegetables such as potatoes, parsnips, and corn are also excluded or greatly minimized in these diets.

The reduced fiber in such diets can cause many to suffer from constipation. Dietary fiber is required for proper digestion and metabolism. Most people I know on these diets need help with laxatives. We should eat balanced meals consisting of a variety of good quality fats, good quality carbs, which can be vegetables, fruits, grains, etc., (Let me emphasize here that healthy carbs should not be demonized) good quality proteins, and drink plenty of water.

This is the best way to make healthy food choices—eating something from many food groups in moderation. What we feed our bodies should be enough to make our bodies work efficiently and unaided.

## Meals with a High Fat Content

I have looked at many Keto Diet recipes, and I find the fat content of many of the suggested meals alarming, as do many health experts and nutritionists. Again, according to a CNN health article,[13] the very high fat content of this diet typically amounts to 70% of daily calorie intake with carbohydrates amounting to a meager 15- 20% per day. Many of these experts flip the Keto Diet on its side and recommend that 45-65% of daily calories should come from carbs, 20-35% from total fats, with less than 10% from saturated fat, and 10-35% of calories should be protein based. Also, I cannot help but wonder what potential side effects a long-term, high-fat diet might have on an otherwise healthy individual.

## Low-Carb Meals

Prolonged low-carb diets can potentially be dangerous, and there really are no studies proving their safety. In the past, I have tried to heavily restrict carbs in my diet and always ended up with raging headaches. I know someone who had fainting spells probably because of insufficient carbs. I honestly do not know how anyone can sustain a severely reduced or no-carb diet.

## Complex Food Planning

I personally think that some of these diets require rather complex food preparations. Daily food planning and eating does not have to be so elaborate. It certainly should not be a daunting experience. Generally, the world's food system is unnecessarily complicated, with too many fad diets in the mix.[14] In my opinion, the reintroduction phase in the whole-30 plan discussed above would be tricky to implement. This would certainly be a deal breaker for me.

We will do well to eat primarily from the nutritious foods that God has blessed us with in moderation. They are generally quite easy to prepare.

## Food Taste

I also can only imagine that the taste of low- and no-carb breads and pizza crusts, etc., used in many diets, leave a lot to be desired, as do the tastes of most low-calorie, store-bought packaged meals. They really are not very tasty. My experience with them in the past was that they had to be doctored up to be remotely tasty. By this I mean various spices and other ingredients have to be added to these foods to make them more palatable. So why bother? Our meals will be more enjoyable if they are made from real, nutrient-dense ingredients. I see no harm in occasionally having a sensible portion of pizza or bread, preferably the whole grain variety, and other foods that we enjoy.

## Successful Weight Loss and Maintenance

I truly believe that most weight loss diets are often an unpleasant experience, primarily because they are overly restrictive, causing participants to crave "forbidden" foods. In my opinion, being deprived of many foods, especially those that we would typically eat and enjoy outside the strict rules of a diet, can very well lead to anxiety and crankiness. That was certainly my experience, and I had headaches too. These diets seldom result in desired permanent weight loss, anyway. Often, weight is initially lost and quickly regained, usually with extra pounds, after heavily restricted diets. For the most part, these diets are cumbersome and unsustainable. Eating does not have to be so. These types of diets are not the answer.

You are probably now thinking: How can I lose the weight I want or need to? Let me tell you how. I will start by saying that many people want to lose weight quickly--often too quickly. However, rapid weight loss is usually caused by severely limiting diets that allow very little food. This manner of weight loss is often difficult to maintain. The most efficient way for successful weight loss/maintenance is by forming healthy eating habits. This will involve engaging our minds as we eat,[15] and incorporating a wide variety of nutrient-dense foods, in our meals. These foods are healthy and nourishing and energizing. (I explain this further in Chapter 3). With this approach, we are less likely to have food cravings, and we will probably better enjoy our food, too. That has been my experience.

We can achieve our goals by choosing primarily healthy foods and eating them in moderation. Good eating is the main component for a healthy lifestyle--say about 80%. The balance of 20% is exercise. We need to exercise moderately, too. In other words, we should strive to make moderate healthy eating and exercise a part of our lifestyle. It really is that simple.

This is how I lost my excess weight and have kept it off for close to three decades. It was not a dramatic weight loss. It happened slowly over about a year. In Chapter 4, I discuss briefly how I ate in order to lose weight. In Chapter 8, I discuss the role of exercise in our healthy lifestyle pursuit. Barring various conditions, some of which I discuss in Chapter 10, this method should work for you, too.

I cannot overemphasize that moderately fueling our bodies with a wide variety of healthy foods is essential to long-term weight loss and maintenance.

# Chapter 3

# God's Way

Now let us look at eating the way God intended us to. For anyone thinking, "Does God really care about what we eat?" Yes, He does. Indeed, He cares about all facets of our lives. We are the apple of His eye. He knows even the number of hairs on our head.

**Luke 12:7 KJV**

*But even the very hairs of your head are all numbered...*

As God is caring enough to have knowledge of the number of our hairs, it is very reasonable to believe that He must also care about what we eat. Indeed, He loves us so much and has a very keen interest inall that concerns us.

We have already established in Chapter 1 that our bodies are His temple. He wants His temple well-fed and well looked after. Yes, God is very interested in what we eat. He addressed this very early in His Word:

**Genesis 1:29 AMPC**
*And God said, See, I have given you every plant yielding seed that is on the face of all the land and every tree with seed in its fruit; you shall have them for food.*

**Genesis 2:16 KJV**
*And the Lord God commanded the man, saying, of every tree of the garden thou mayest freely eat.*

He did not bless us with so many different plants as food only for us to eat a very limited variety, avoiding so many fruits and veggies as suggested by some fad diets and expectlong-termsuccess with our weight loss/maintenance goals.

## How About Meat?

Scripture tells us that in the beginning people ate only plants. It was after the great flood that the eating of meat was first mentioned.

**Genesis 9:3 KJV**
*Every moving thing that liveth shall be meat for you; even as the green herb have I given you all things.*

**Psalms 103:5 KJV**
*Who satisfieth thy mouth with good things; so that thy youth is renewed like the eagle's.*

Our good God wants us well-nourished with food so that we are fit and strong to fulfill His purpose for our lives. It is not eating moderately the foods that God has so graciously provided us that ails us. It is all the overly pro-cessed foods, snacks, and drinks eaten regularly and often excessively by many that is the problem. I discuss this in more detail in Chapter 5.

**Ecclesiastes 3:13 NLT**
*And people should eat and drink and enjoy the fruits of their labor, for these are gifts from God.*

**Ecclesiastes 5:18 KJV**
*Behold that which I have seen: it is good and comely for one to eat and to drink, and to enjoy the good of all his labour that he taketh under the sun all the days of his life, which God giveth him: for it is his portion.*

Let us look at the foods that God has provided us. These foods are high in nutrients and relatively low in cal-ories. They are nutrient-dense foods that contain vitamins, minerals, complex carbohydrates, lean protein, and healthy fats.[1] They are essentially good quality carbs, good quality proteins, and good quality fats. These are all very healthy and nutritious foods that are best consumed when minimally processed. They typically provide a ton of hunger-curbing fiber and more nutrition bang for the calorie buck.[2] Many of these can be eaten close to how they grow in nature, with minimum processing. They are also best grown the way that God intended.[3] The importance of healthy farming practices is discussed later in this chapter.

## What Are Good-Quality Carbs?

Good-quality carbohydrates (carbs) are vegetables (veggies), fruits, legumes, beans, and whole grains. Whole grains are the best source of this group of foods, providing energy, vitamins, minerals and fiber.[4] They can be high or low in carbs. Many weight-loss diets demonize carbs, labelling them as foods to be avoided. This can be very misleading, as many foods rich in carbs are necessary for a healthy diet.[5] There is nothing wrong with carbs in your diet. It is their quality that matters.[6] Not all carb-rich foods are created equal. High-quality carbs consist of essential vitamins, minerals, nutrients and fiber. The fiber helps control fluctuations in blood sugar and insulin; they slow down the digestion of sugars and starches, thus preventing large spikes in these two compounds. When these levels are high and uncontrolled, they can contribute to chronic illnesses such as diabetes, heart disease, and overeating, resulting in weight gain. In addition, elevated insulin levels cause our cells to become resistant to the hormone insulin. Fiber also ensures regular bowel movements, which are essential for good health.

Examples of these high fiber carbs are veggies like sweet potatoes, tomatoes, mushrooms, carrots, mixed greens, kale, spinach, Brussels sprouts, artichokes, and squash. Other examples are legumes such as kidney beans, black beans, and lentils, and grains such as whole grain breads, brown rice, pasta, quinoa, and barley. Also, fruits like papaya, mangoes, oranges, pineapples, peaches, apples, pears, and berries. These are all healthy, and we will do our bodies well to eat a variety of them in moderation. A useful tip is to have smaller portions of fruits with a high sugar content, like grapes, mangoes, and pineapples.

## Good-Quality Proteins

Proteins are a vital nutrient, required for building, maintaining, and repairing tissues, cells, and organs throughout the body. When we eat protein, it is broken down into 20 amino acids. These are the basic building blocks of the body for growth and energy. Protein energizes the body and supports our mood and cognitive functions.[7]

Many animal sources of protein, such as poultry, eggs, meat, dairy, and fish, deliver all the amino acids our bodies need. Protein sources from plants such as vegetables, grains, beans, and nuts often lack one or more of the essential amino acids.[8]

Proteins can be low or high quality. For good health, we should eat the latter variety. Typically, high-quality sources of animal protein are organic, grass-fed, and are minimally processed when ready for consumption. Conversely, low-quality sources are industrially raised meats that are often highly processed before consumption.[9]

Some processed meats, for example, corned beef and cold cuts, contain significant amounts of protein; however, many are loaded with various additives and salt which can elevate blood pressure. According to a BBC News article, "Processed meats do cause cancer - WHO," by James Gallagher, 26 October 2015, these meats have also been linked to an increased risk of some cancers.

**What are the health benefits of high-quality proteins?**[10]

- They give us the energy to get up and go.

- They are vital for maintaining our health as we age.

- Helps our body repair itself after injury.

- Helps increase fat burning, by boosting our metabolism.

- They may help curb our appetite by making us feel full longer, and thus help maintain a healthy weight.

- Fuels us with extra energy for exercising.

- Helps us think clearly and may improve our memory.

- They are good for our bones.

- Helps us maintain healthy skin, hair, and nails.

- Helps increase muscle mass.

We should try to divide our protein intake equally among meals. We also need to be mindful of our individual health conditions. For example, too much protein may be harmful for people with kidney disease.

## What are Good-Quality Sources of Protein?[11]

### Poultry

Organic and free-range poultry is best, as the non-organic birds may contain antibiotics and are likely to have been raised on GMO feed that was also treated with pesticides.[12] Removing the skin from chicken and turkey before consumption can substantially reduce the saturated fat content of a meal.

## Fish

Typically, seafood is high in protein and low in saturated fat. Varieties such as sardines, salmon, trout, anchovies, and herring are also high in omega-3 fatty acids. It is recommended that we eat seafood at least twice a week.[13]

## Legumes

These are a type of vegetable that includes beans, lentils, peanuts, and peas. This group of foods is both versatile and nutritious and packed full of protein and fiber. They can be added to salads, soups, and stews to boost the fiber and protein content in these foods. Other than peanuts, they are low in fat, high in potassium, magnesium, iron, and folate.[14]

## Nuts and Seeds

Nuts and seeds are rich sources of protein. They are also high in "good" fats and fiber. They too make a delicious addition to salads. Nuts are a particularly handy, nutritious snack, especially when out and about.[15]

## What are Good Quality Fats?[16]

Not all fats are healthy. Fats are mainly saturated or unsaturated. A diet high in saturated fats can raise cholesterol levels, and therefore increase the risk of heart disease and stroke. Healthy dietary fats are mostly unsaturated. These fats can be either monounsaturated or polyunsaturated. They both help in reducing the levels of bad LDL cholesterol. In addition, monounsaturated fats help protect our hearts by maintaining levels of good HDL cholesterol.

Monounsaturated or polyunsaturated fats are good quality fats. They are found in a variety of foods and oils and are best consumed in their purest form and as close to how they appear in nature. Monounsaturated fats are found in nuts and oils.

The two main types of polyunsaturated fats are omega-3 and omega-6.

Omega-3 fats are found in oily fish like:

- Sardines

- Salmon

- Kippers

- Mackerel

Whether vegetable sources of omega-3 fats have the same benefits on heart health as those found in fish is still controversial.[17]

Omega-6 fats are found in vegetable oils like:

- Corn

- Sunflower

- Rapeseed and in some nuts

It is not a good idea to overheat oils when we cook. A study in the Canadian Journal of Dietetic Practice and Research found that when oils are heated to smoking point, the amount of polyunsaturated fatty acids are reduced because of oxidative degradation. This brings about a loss of some of their nutritional benefits.[18]

We typically get enough omega-6 in our diet. To ensure adequate levels of omega-3 we should eat at least two portions of fish each week, one being an oily fish.

God has blessed us all with a wide variety of healthy foods. The most nutritious and delicious foods readily available will be closely related to the part of the world that we live in. Therefore, if we live in areas where mangoes or kiwi fruits are grown, we will enjoy more nutritious and delicious mangoes and kiwi fruits than those who live far away from these areas.[19]

Typically, fruits exported around the world are plucked before they are ripe, with the ripening process continuing as they are transported across the globe. These fruits are less nutritious and not nearly as delicious as those allowed to ripen before they are picked, sold, and consumed near their source. There is nothing like fruit in season that has been allowed to tree-ripen before they are plucked. They burst with flavor and are at their best nutritionally.[20]

God has graciously blessed us with good quality foods (crops and animals). Poor farming practices will affect the quality of these foods. The best crops are grown on land grazed by free, roaming farm animals. They ensure that the soil is naturally fertilized with their droppings.[21]

Animals raised in concentrated feeding systems are typically fed abnormal foods, not what they would naturally eat. They are often given hormones to fatten them up. These animals end up quite sick and are often given various antibiotics, which eventually are consumed by us when we eat them. Never forget that we end up eating what the animals we eat have ingested.[22]

We will do well to include moderate amounts of these high-quality foods in our daily meals. They have been graciously provided by our good God and should be eaten and enjoyed in moderation. He loves us and wants us to enjoy these foods.

# Chapter 4

# My Way

I am now going to walk you through the way of eating that has worked for me. I am not promising fast results but a sustainable way of eating and maintaining weight loss. What I will do is show you a systematic approach to changing your eating habits. Ultimately, my plan is to get you to lose weight and keep it off...let's relegate yo-yo dieting to our past.

Very briefly, yo-yo dieting[1] refers to a pattern of losing weight, regaining it, and then trying to lose it again. There is nothing beneficial about this way of dieting. It can have a negative impact on our body fat percentage at the expense of muscle mass and strength. This is discussed further in *Chapter 7*. Yo-yo dieting can also cause fatty liver disease, high blood pressure, diabetes, and heart disease. It is best to make small, permanent lifestyle changes. Let me show you how.

I have maintained my weight for over 25 years, by making healthy food choices, primarily from nutrient dense foods; and eating out of these, a good variety of foods that I enjoy. I am quite adventurous. My food choices are generally influenced by my location. I spent a lot of time in Nigeria, the country of my birth as I wrote this book, so many of the foods that I mention in this chapter are native to Nigeria.

I am always eager to explore new foods and I do when I travel. I also mention a few of these foods I have enjoyed in this chapter.

I share at the end of this chapter, a list of many of the highly nutritious foods that I include in my meals. To eat well, it is best to choose a mix of similar foods available where you are every day.

I like to call this approach to food The Moderate Approach to Food. I generally do not like the term "diet," as it usually refers to eating sparingly, often with a feeling of deprivation. I believe it is possible to lose and maintain weight loss without feeling deprived. The key to sustaining good eating habits is to begin by planning with healthy foods in our pantry.[2] By planning, I mean having an idea what we will eat *before* mealtimes. We set ourselves up to fail if we do not plan our meals and try to figure out what to eat, especially when we are hungry.

When our meals are not planned, we are likely to pick at food erratically and maybe even binge. This is a good reason why we should buy and store mainly healthy foods. As much as possible, we should also avoid grocery shopping when we are hungry. When we do, we are likely to end up buying much more food than is needed. Also, have you seen people in grocery stores, indiscriminately eating all the food samples that are available? Or opening and eating from snack packets as they fill their baskets/trolleys before they are paid for? I have. I imagine the main reason for these actions is hunger. We should always try to write a well-thought-out shopping list beforehand and stick to it.

We must learn to look beyond the well-stacked confectionery, crisps, and fizzy drinks aisles in grocery stores.[3]Let's start to get acquainted with the aisles where real, fresh foods are stacked. Beware of the craftily placed chocolate bars and other tempting items by checkout counters. Where available, we should patronize the fast-growing health food industry. These foods may not be cheap, but it is money spent well for better nutrition. It is an investment in our health. It is better, and cheaper in the long run, to spend it there than on hospital bills. Prevention is always better than cure.

If we do not have a pantry stashed with unhealthy foods and snacks, we will not have easy access to them. Our food plans should be based on the healthy foods and drinks we enjoy, avoiding overly processed foods, which are often loaded with sugar, and therefore contain empty calories. These foods are discussed extensively in the next chapter. Empty calories are derived from various high processed foods and beverages; they contain no nutrients. A good example is refined sugar.

Now let's take a look at our meals. I recommend at least three meals a day. Typically, we should make the veggie portion of our meals substantial, the protein portion adequate, and carbs minimal. I tend to have a good breakfast. I believe that it is a very important meal and sets the tone for the rest of our day. It gives us the energy required for our various daily activities both physical and mental. Lunch is generally my biggest meal and dinner my smallest. There is a lot to be said about the size of our meals and when we eat them. Eating the bulk of our food early in the day gives our bodies time to convert food to energy and utilize it for various activities as opposed to storing it as fat.

I have a variety of foods I choose from at breakfast. I start my day with water and a small amount of fruit. My choice will depend on what is in season and where I am in the world. This is sometimes followed by an omelette made with two egg whites and sardines, or with cheddar cheese and spinach, and a cup of decaf coffee or herbal tea. I eat egg white omelettes only because I do not like the taste or smell of egg yolks. I will often add a couple of medium slices of almond bread or any other multi-grain brown bread on days that I exercise.

A recent breakfast option I have added is oatmeal cooked in water, to which I add unsweetened crunchy peanut butter and a small chopped banana. A breakfast meal I enjoy on a strenuous workout day is **akara**, a sort of fritter made from black-eyed beans native to Brazil and parts of Africa. Occasionally I will have some pap with it. Pap is made from dry white or yellow corn and has a distinct sour taste. It has the consistency of custard or grits. It can be eaten on its own or as an accompaniment. This is quite a heavy meal and is very welcome, as I am often famished after a rigorous workout, particularly when it is first thing in the morning.

On a day when I do not intend to exercise, I will eat a breakfast of fruit, **moimoi** (a Nigerian steamed bean pudding made from a mixture of washed, peeled and ground black-eyed beans, onions, fresh ground red peppers and salt), or an egg white omelette with veggies such as sweet peppers, mushrooms, cauliflower, or broccoli. Alternatively, I might have a plain egg white omelette with a few pieces of avocado pear and a cup of decaf coffee or herbal tea. On these days, I usually do not have pap or bread, as they both have more carbs than I care to consume on an exercise-free day.

I like my lunch plate to be colorful when eating "continental style." I could have roasted meat or fish with at least two or three different veggies. Depending on where I am in the world, my veggie choices vary. I tend to choose from mushrooms, broccoli, cabbage, sweet peppers, beetroot, carrots, parsnips, cauliflower, and some greens such as spinach, kale, or other locally grown greens readily available in Nigeria and a small portion of carbs. I like my vegetables sautéed lightly with olive oil or other healthy oils, roasted, or lightly steamed.

Let me interject here for clarity that veggies contain carbs. I use the term carbs in *small portion of carbs* in the paragraph above, specifically in relation to other carbs. These include brown pasta or rice, quinoa, baked or fried sweet potatoes, and plantains, which I have either boiled, roasted, or fried.

My meat choices can be beef, goat, chicken, Guinea fowl or lamb. Here again my choices will be influenced by location. On a day when I have exercised hard, I may even indulge in a dessert. A small portion is sufficient and very satisfying. It keeps me from feeling deprived.

When I eat Nigerian food at lunch, it consists of a lot of vegetable soup and meat or fish and a small portion of carbs. I am big on vegetables, and there is a variety of delicious Nigerian vegetable soups from which to choose. I am not too keen on what is now popularly known as "swallow" in Nigerian parlance.

This is typically high in carbohydrates and can be made from a wide variety of carbohydrates, like, yam, plantain, ground rice, oatmeal, etc. It is somewhat similar to mashed potatoes, but not as fluffy...it is heavier. It is always accompanied by one of the many Nigerian soups. These foods are called swallow as they are typically eating without being chewed. When I do eat any of these, it is usually no bigger than the size of my fist. I do not eat these foods more than ten times a year, as I prefer other carbohydrates like slightly ripe plantain roasted or boiled, and sometimes fried ripe plantain, roasted cocoyam (a tropical root vegetable), and boiled or roasted sweet potatoes with Nigerian vegetable soups.

Occasionally, I will eat a small portion of rice, usually *ofada* (a minimally processed rice blend), with some fried plantain and vegetable soup. I also eat and enjoy a plate of beans with fried, boiled, or roasted plantain, again with a side portion of a Nigerian vegetable soup. I eat this at least a couple of times per month. Another Nigerian meal I occasionally enjoy at lunchtime is yam or sweet potato pottage (yam or sweet potato cooked in a thick soup or stew) with vegetables. I always eat a good portion of vegetable soup or sautéed vegetables whenever I eat Nigerian food at lunch. I must have something green on my plate...bring on the veggies! This is atypical, as it is not uncommon for many in Nigeria to eat a plate of, say, rice and chicken stew without any vegetables.

You are probably thinking: How I can eat all these carbs and not be overweight? I now have a high metabolism. However, I was overweight up until my late twenties, when I got a grip and radically changed the way I ate and started to exercise. I dropped; 6-8 dress sizes, and I have kept it off for nearly 30 years. Unfortunately, I can't tell you how much weight I lost. I have always preferred to keep tabs on my weight using the way my clothes fit me. I have no doubt in my mind that if I did not make drastic changes to my lifestyle, which also helped increase my metabolism, I would have remained that way or more likely grown bigger.

My new lifestyle, which includes eating nutrient-dense foods and an exercise regimen, has greatly improved my metabolism. A "high" metabolism means more calories are required to maintain weight. On the other hand, a person with a "low" (or slow) metabolism will burn fewer calories at rest and during activity, and therefore have to eat less to avoid becoming overweight. I discuss metabolism in more detail in *Chapter 7*.

If you continue to read carefully, you will see that even though I eat carbs, I do keep a close eye on their quality. Not all carbs are created equal.[4] As I keep saying, moderation is key...please stay with me. You must have heard of that popular saying, "Breakfast like a king, lunch like a prince, eat dinner like a pauper." I practice a slight variation: I breakfast like a prince, lunch like a king, and eat dinner like a pauper.

At dinner, I typically eat veggies and grilled chicken or fish, or steamed fish. Sometimes I may have a bowl of pepper soup with chicken or fish, often with a side salad. Some evenings I will have a vegetable smoothie, sometimes with a low sugar fruit added. Notice the minimal carbs? I am super cautious with carbs after 4 p.m. I heard of this tactic from Jada Pinkett-Smith, a Black-American actress, who mentioned that it worked for her. In my opinion, she looks good, so I was keen to pay attention to her tips.

Now remember that there are exceptions to every rule. I will occasionally eat carbs for dinner. At these times, I am very mindful that I will not be exerting myself too much before bedtime and will very often be careful the following day. Another rule I have with dinner is not to have it late. I am usually done eating before 7 p.m. I truly believe that we should endeavor not to eat too late and, when we do, we should be extra careful as we are typically less active at night.

Strictly adhering to this rule played a tremendous role in ensuring that my excess weight was lost, and it has helped me maintain my reduced weight over the years. I have not eaten late consistently for close to 30 years, and so now find it quite uncomfortable when I do. This is an added incentive for me not to eat late. My close family and friends all know that this is a principle that I am strict about. I believe that our bodies do not like drama. They prefer a structured approach to eating and indeed to most aspects of our lives.

## Do You Get Home Late?

For people who work late or are not able to arrive home early enough to eat before 7 p.m., I strongly advise that you choose foods that will not cause havoc to your waistline. These will typically be high in protein, low sugar, and low GI (Glycemic Index) foods,[5] such as lean meats chicken or fish) and lots of low-carb cooked veggies, or a fresh salad made with low-carb veggies. These will not cause your blood sugar levels to spike. The effects of this are discussed in the next paragraph. Try to eat the carbs your body needs, and I dare say craves, at breakfast and lunch.

Perhaps you can take a packed lunch to work with protein, healthy carbs, and veggies. Most companies provide a microwave oven for staff. Otherwise learn to make and eat healthy choices from foods provided in the canteen or at nearby eateries.

Loading down on carbs in the evening, especially late, equates to trouble...weight gain. This is especially true if one is sedentary after a high-carb meal and goes to bed soon after. When carb rich foods are eaten, our blood sugar can rise. With minimal movement as we get ready for bed, it can remain heightened until the following morning. If more carbs are consumed at breakfast, one's blood can really get loaded with sugar. As our levels of blood sugar rise, the pancreas produces insulin. This hormone prompts cells to absorb blood sugar for energy or storage, causing a blood sugar dip (helping control the amount of sugar (glucose) in the blood). Some people are resistant to the hormone insulin, resulting in an increase in their blood sugar. With insulin resistance, the body's cells do not respond normally to insulin. This can result in glucose not entering the cells as easily, and so causing a build-up in the blood, which can eventually lead to type 2 diabetes. This condition is discussed in further detail in **Chapter 10**.

A healthy watch should be placed over carbs, but there is no need for them to be demonized, as they often are in many fad weight loss diets. There is nothing wrong with eating moderate amounts of good quality carbs. These were discussed in detail in **Chapter 3**.

My plan as I have described above is based on what I enjoy eating. It is obviously more extensive than I have shared, as I am not generally a fussy eater. I enjoy a wide array of healthy foods. My moderate approach to food helps me maintain my weight. We keep a healthy check on our weight when we keep it stable, with fluctuations of no more than a kilogram or two either way. I have pretty much eaten this way for over 25 years, and my weight has not fluctuated much. I developed a healthy relationship with food by eating this way. Comfort eating became a habit of my past. I quickly had reduced cravings, particularly for processed sugar, other unhealthy carbs and fats, indeed all unhealthy foods. A healthy relationship with food curbs food binges, as we learn to eat what we enjoy in moderation.

When we eat mindfully,[6] we instinctively know that if we have had a couple of days of indulgent eating, we are somewhat careful the next few days and get back into a healthy. moderate eating pattern. Trust me, eating this way also makes meals more enjoyable and satisfying, too.

## When Should We Stop Eating?

It is wise to keep a watchful eye on the amount of food we eat. When we do not, we can eat mindlessly--not paying adequate attention to what and how much is consumed. Mindless eaters often eat with their eyes and not their stomach. They tend to get carried away with all that is available to them, without much regard to what they can consume comfortably.[7] When we eat this way, we often end up eating way too much. We will do ourselves good to be more conscious about what we eat and the quantity we eat.

When at home, we can help ourselves to be more mindful about what we eat by working on our environment. Stocking our pantries with healthy food choices is a wise move. As mentioned above, to achieve this, it is not a good idea to go shopping when hungry. When we do, we are likely to purchase much more food than is required and buy unhealthy snacks for a quick fix.

Eating healthy portions is as important as eating the right foods. Moderation is key, even when we are eating healthy. We should never gorge ourselves on food.[8] When we do, we are likely to be uncomfortable, and this can cause stress to our digestive system. Typically, I like to have a plate with a lot of vegetables, a good portion of protein, and a small portion of good quality carbs. I tend to put appropriate amounts I know I can eat on my plate. I have developed a good sense over the years of what is enough food for me. If I finish it and feel like I want more, I will often wait a while—say, five minutes. More often than not, I will find that I have had enough. If I still feel the need for more food after five minutes, I may drink more water and, if the desire persists, I will eat some more protein and vegetables, usually smaller portions than my original helping.

Sometimes, particularly on a day when I have exercised, I will have a dessert. This is never excessive. At this point, I have already eaten a good meal anyway; therefore, not much more food is needed for me to feel satisfied. This scenario will usually take place at lunch, as it is at this time that I eat the most. Remember the rule of eating dinner like a pauper. Of course, there are exceptions to the rule, just do not let the exception occur too often. I have learned to work daily at not being overfed and undernourished.[9] This is quite easy to achieve when we make healthy food choices.

### The French Approach to Food[10]

In researching this book, I decided to look at the French and their approach to food. Why is it that in the land of cheese, butter, cream, and croissants the French are generally quite slim? They enjoy their meals, eat a wide variety of foods, and eat well. Allow me to quickly interject here...with real butter, a thin spread is sufficient to enjoy its delicious taste. My opinion regarding the various butter spreads, is that they never taste right.

The French tend to have a healthy relationship with food that was taught in their childhood. This includes learning to sit at a table, eat a wide variety of foods, and enjoy eating in an unhurried, sociable manner. As has been mentioned before, we must eat to survive, so we will do well acquiring a healthy relationship with food early in life. This will involve us eating a wide variety of healthy foods and learning to know when to stop.

The French also pay attention to their food presentation. I think that eating a well-presented meal is far more appealing, and therefore better enjoyed, than one that is served haphazardly on our plate. The French eat a good balance of a variety of mostly healthy foods. The diverse variety of foods helps to ensure that they do not get bored with their meals. Eating appears to be a very conscious process for them.

Many French foods can be quite rich, but it does not appear to have an adverse effect on their weight. I believe this is because they eat these rich foods in moderation, balanced with lots of fruits and veggies, which can be raw or cooked as a portion of the meal, and as a soup or in a smoothie.

As we well know, the French do eat a lot of baguettes, a type of French bread. These do not contain added sugar as is often the case with bread in the US and other countries. This is probably one reason why their waistlines are unaffected. They seem to eat a lot of everything but not too much of anything. The French typically do not diet, so they do not eat low fat, fat free, low sugar manufactured diet foods, as most other nationalities tend to do. These diet products are often ultra-processed. The French are also unlikely to eliminate entire food groups from their meals. They do not have a culture of eating processed foods, and they manage their meal portions. They avoid GM (genetically modified) foods like the plague.

As they eat everything in moderation, they seldom get uncontrollable cravings. In my opinion, this is one of the biggest causes of failures in eating plans. The French tend not to wait until they are starving and typically do not eat too much. They regularly eat home cooked meals prepared with fresh produce bought from the farmers market whenever possible. They do eat desserts, chocolates, and other confectionaries as evidenced by their numerous *patisseries*. Apparently, they indulge wisely and not as much as you would think, and certainly not as many movies suggest. They also do not have a culture of fizzy drinks, which are often quite sweet--all "food for thought." They tend not to drink excessive amounts of alcohol. They will occasionally enjoy a glass of wine with their meal. They take the time to appreciate the taste of the different ingredients and textures in their food. When you are mindful of what you eat, you instinctively know when you are full. You stop then and are less likely to overeat. Moderation is key, seems to be their motto. They have truly mastered the art of paying attention to what they eat. My approach to food is very similar to that of the French.

It really is worthwhile teaching children how to eat well and develop a healthy relationship with food early in life. French children are taught at school to sit and eat up to four courses at the age of 2-4. Teach them young and they are likely to retain good habits throughout their lives.

## My Eating Habits Pre-Weight Loss

I want to include here very briefly how I ate prior to losing weight. When I look back to those years, I can see why I was overweight. I had no cognizance whatsoever of the different food groups or much, if any, knowledge of a balanced diet. I would often eat packets of crisps, biscuits, and chocolate bars for a meal with a can of Coke or any other sugar-laden beverage that took my fancy. In addition, it was not uncommon for me to snack on these high-sugar items well into the night. These awful eating habits were heightened if I was feeling unhappy or going through a difficult time.

## What I Did to Lose Weight

Prior to my maintenance eating plan, I went on a weight loss eating regime. I had been overweight in my teenage years and well into my twenties.

To lose weight, we must eat less and be more active. Losing weight is one thing. Keeping it off is another matter entirely. The main variation in my weight loss eating plan and the way I eat now, and have for nearly 30 years, is in my portion sizes. Some may benefit from using a smaller plate in the weight loss phase, as it may help control portion sizes. I was also very particular about the carbs I ate in that phase; I also consumed more proteins, vegetables and always chose low sugar fruits.

It was at this time that I started to incorporate exercise into my lifestyle. My routines have evolved over the years. There will be more discussion on the role of exercise in developing and maintaining a healthy lifestyle in Chapter 8.

I did not have the relationship I now have with the Lord when I lost weight those many years ago. At that time, I did not know to depend totally on the Lord for guidance in all things as I do now. I am convinced that my weight loss journey would have been easier and with fewer setbacks. I discuss in **Chapter 11** how God's Word can help us achieve our weight loss/maintenance goals.

I am available to discuss and walk you through this essential, initial part of your journey to eating well for a paid consultation. I can be contacted at **owen@eatandexercisehealthy.com** I am not promising a drastic change in your weight, but a gradual and steady weight loss, and a wholesome relationship with food providing my instructions are followed. Barring any unforeseen conditions, such as those discussed in Chapter 10, and others that I have not covered, my plan truly ensures weight loss and its maintenance.

## How I Eat Now

I now have a very healthy relationship with food and really enjoy my meals. I also am quite strict about my eating times. I pretty much eat at the same time daily. I find that having an eating routine helps me to be very much in tune with my body. I never get too hungry and do not stuff myself when I eat.

We are what we eat. We should make healthy food choices from good proteins, good carbs, and good fats. Eat a variety of all the different foods that we like from these choices in moderation and drink plenty of water. When we eat healthy in combination with a good exercise regime, we will more than likely lose weight, keep it off, and enjoy a healthy lifestyle.

These are some of the nutrient dense foods I enjoy:

- Oily fish such as salmon, trout, and sardines

- Chicken which is a cheap and healthy meat

- Guinea fowl

- Kale—possibly the most nutritious of all leafy green vegetables

- Spinach and other leafy green vegetables available where you live

- Avocado

- Plantains

- Coco yam

- Sweet potatoes

- Egg whites

- Garlic—a nutritious vegetable considered part of the onion family and may boost immune function[11]

- Broccoli

- Quinoa

- Beetroot

- Oats

- Legumes and nuts

- Blackberries and blueberries

- Seasonal fruits and vegetables--as available

When we consciously choose from and eat more of these types of foods, we will get the beneficial nutrients our body needs without consuming too many calories. These foods have a very high nutrient content relative to the number of calories that they contain.[12]

Eating primarily nutrient-dense foods, keeping a watch on the quantities I ate, and on my mealtimes, helped me lose my excess weight. I have kept the weight off by continuing to eat this way. It can work for you, too.

# Chapter 5

# Processed Sugar, Foods, and Drinks

We live in a world that offers a proliferation of overly processed foods and drinks. Many of these processed items contain refined sugar and/or hydrogenated fats and salt. I will use the terms processed, refined sugar, overly processed, highly processed, and processed foods interchangeably. Let's take a look at the main culprits in processed foods.

## Processed Sugar

There are copious quantities of this sugar in popular highly processed foods and drinks such as cakes, biscuits, muffins, pies, breads, and seemingly healthy foods like high fiber breakfast cereals and various sugar-laden beverages. Unfortunately, the high amount of sugars in these foods has largely been overlooked by the public health establishment's obsession with fat.[1]

There is now enough evidence to prove that sugar is a bigger "demon" than fat for people seeking weight loss and maintenance. As discussed in Chapter 2, there are high fat diets which cause weight loss. Clearly, fat does not necessarily preclude weight loss. Typically, these diets are totally void of processed carbs and allow only minuscule amounts of healthy carbs. Remember though, as discussed in Chapter 2, these diets are unlikely to be sustainable long-term and are perhaps better used to jumpstart a weight loss program or get back on track after a period of indulgence. One thing that these diets do prove emphatically is that, despite their lack of sustainability, the consumption of fat does not stop us from losing weight. It is processed sugar and other unhealthy carbs that we should keep an extra vigilant eye on in our quest for weight loss and maintenance.

There are copious amounts of refined sugar in many processed foods.[2] I pretty much demonize this sugar, as it can add unnecessary, unwanted calories—the so-called empty calories. We have got to be super vigilant in keeping tabs on refined sugar calories; they are not only empty but can negatively affect our weight reduction plans and also cause havoc to our waistline when we are in the maintenance phase.

Case in point: I had a procedure that required a significant increase in my water consumption. To make it easier, I often added Ribena (usually a blackcurrant concentrate) to my water. About three to four months later, I noticed that my waistline had thickened. I instinctively knew that Ribena was the culprit, as it was the only newly added item. Thankfully, I lost the few extra pounds quickly when I stopped drinking Ribena. I then used fresh lemon and other fresh fruit juices to flavor my water.

What struck me was how the extra weight disappeared after I stopped adding Ribena to my water. It was alarming to me, because I had only added small amounts, and so thought that all was well. This just goes to show you the dangers of processed sugar.

I have another Ribena story. My sister used to be a fan and drank it daily. She was cautious and made sure she only added a small amount to her water. She found out at a dental appointment that the enamel on her front teeth was being affected. She replaced Ribena with plain water. Guess what happened? She quickly lost weight around her mid-section. She had no idea, prior to her decision to stop, the effect it was having on her weight. My take from this is that we must also beware of citric acid as it can erode the enamel in our teeth, when consumed excessively. This makes our teeth more susceptible to decay. Looks like the safest drink is the elixir of life...water.

Refined sugars can do more harm to our bodies than an increase of our waistlines and body weight. There will be further discussion on the negative impact of processed sugar, foods, and drinks later in this chapter. I also include a further discussion of these sugars, specifically high fructose corn syrup.

## Salt

Salt is one of the ubiquitous ingredients found in overly processed foods. It is often found in many products that you may not expect it to be present in, such as breakfast cereals, cakes, chocolate bars, biscuits, dessert pastries, and bread.

When we eat too much salt, extra water is stored in our bodies, which causes our blood pressure to rise. High blood pressure is often referred to as the silent killer because it typically has no symptoms until it has done significant damage to the heart and arteries. In extreme cases, high blood pressure causes a strain on our heart, arteries, kidneys, and brain. This can lead to heart attacks, strokes, dementia, and kidney disease. As we can see, the many salty processed products can be life-threatening if eaten frequently and in large quantities.

## High Fructose Corn Syrup and Hydrogenated Oils

Two other ingredients to keep a close eye on in processed food packaging labels are High Fructose Corn Syrup (HFCS) and Hydrogenated Oil (sometimes listed as partially hydrogenated oil). HFCS was first introduced into foods in America in the 1970s at about the same time as partially hydrogenated oils. Since then, there have been epidemic levels of obesity and other diseases, and reduced life expectancy. This is not a coincidence.[3] These two ingredients are ubiquitous and really should not be consumed at all or at least in very limited amounts.

HFCS is a sweetener derived from corn syrup, which is processed from corn. It is a blend of fructose and glucose: 42% fructose and 58% glucose. In America, where so much corn is grown and is cheaply sourced, food companies tend to use HFCS instead of cane sugar. A big problem with HFCS is that it can be found in many sweetened products like candies, fizzy drinks, and desserts. It is also present in products you would not expect like ketchup, bread, salad dressings, and marinades.[4]

The uncontrolled consumption of these sugars, will cause a spike of insulin in our body and can lead to various health problems. These include weight gain,[5] diabetes, and can even increase the risk of some cancers. Excess fructose that is ingested is readily converted into fat by the liver. Fat stored in the liver can cause a pre-diabetic condition known as Metabolic Syndrome. In summary, metabolic syndrome is a cluster of conditions that occur together that increase the risk of stroke, heart disease, and type 2 diabetes.[6] These conditions include increased blood pressure, high blood sugar, excess body fat around the midsection, and abnormal cholesterol or triglyceride levels. Clearly, we need to watch how much processed sugar we consume. We increase our risk of becoming afflicted with one or more of these ailments if we consume this sugar excessively for sustained periods.

Let's look at Hydrogenated oils.[7] When oils are hydrogenated, they are heated to high temperatures with hydrogen gas added. This process gives food a longer shelf life and results in a product more commonly known as transfats. These fats have been proven to lower our HDL (good cholesterol) levels and raise our LDL (bad cholesterol) levels. These changes are contributory factors to atherosclerosis and coronary heart disease. They can predispose people who consume them indiscriminately to excessive weight gain leading to a struggle with obesity and diabetes.[8]

Regulations in many countries,[9] now require food companies to list the amount of trans-fat on their nutritional labels. The World Health Organization (WHO) has been very involved with the movement to eradicate these fats from the global food-chain. However, WHO only makes recommendations, it will be up to the Governments in various countries to enforce them. Perhaps the results of follow up studies that show a decrease in cardiovascular diseases in countries like Denmark, Switzerland and some states in the US, may encourage others to follow suit.[10] In the US, the FDA has recommended that if the amount is less than half a gram/serving, companies can say, a product contains "zero trans-fat."[11] This can be particularly dangerous as these amounts can add up, if several servings of multiple foods containing these seemingly small amounts are consumed.[12]

Clearly, both partially hydrogenated oils and high fructose corn syrup should be eaten very sparingly and even be deemed "illegal additions to foods."[13] They are *that* deadly when consumed in significant quantities regularly. Unfortunately, the problems associated with trans-fat consumption are not immediate. They cause gradual disease in our body over time. I suspect that if their effect was more spontaneous, they would already be an ingredient of the very distant past. When consumed excessively, over time they can cause chaos from obesity to diabetes to heart disease, etc. These two ingredients are arguably the primary contributing factor for most degenerative diseases.[14] They can increase inflammation, which is associated with an increased risk of obesity, diabetes, and heart disease.

Now let's take a closer look at processed foods and drinks.

## Processed Foods

Generally, food processing refers to the transformation of agricultural produce into food that can be consumed. Some form of food processing is required to make most foods edible and safe. This is referred to as "primary food processing." For example, milk is not sold directly from the cow. It is pasteurized to make it safe for consumption. Secondary food processing converts ingredients into familiar foods. A good example would be the conversion of wheat to bread. Tertiary processed foods have many nutrients stripped and many unhealthy additives introduced.[15] It is this latter type of processed food that I will focus on in this book. Like I mentioned earlier, I use the terms processed, overly processed, and highly processed interchangeably.

Highly processed foods are defined as containing several industrial ingredients such as hydrogenated oils, refined sugar, high-fructose corn syrup, food coloring, flavoring agents, emulsifiers, and various other additives.[16] These foods collectively form what is now popularly known as MAD. This is the acronym for the Modern American Diet.[17]

These cover a wide range of unhealthy foods, which include potato crisps (chips), white rice, various crackers made with white flour, breads (sliced bread, rolls, bagels, and baguettes made with white flour). They also include sugar-sweetened breakfast cereals, microwave popcorn, frozen pizza, store bought biscuits (cookies), and baked goods such as cakes, muffins, and pies,[18] whether they are regular, low-fat, or low-carb. Fast foods, pre-cooked packet meals, etc. are additional examples of overly processed foods.

These foods are typically laden with sugar, sometimes with artificial sweeteners, salt, trans-fats, preservatives, food colorings, other additives, and refined grains. Refined grains are processed with the fiber and other nutrients stripped from them. This is what renders the white color and soft, pillowy texture. Wonder Bread (a brand of bread popular in the US) is well known for this.[19] These processed grains also have a high glycemic Index, which we know means that they can cause our blood sugar levels to spike rapidly.

Consuming too many of these refined foods that often contain a ton of sugar, unhealthy fats, salt and other additives, can eventually lead to metabolic diseases such as diabetes and obesity. To meet our daily intake of gut-healthy fiber and nourish our bodies with the nutrients it needs, we should avoid, or at least severely limit, eating foods made from refined grains and opt for the high fiber variety made from unrefined grains.

## High-Sugar, Carbonated, and Other Drinks

We should also be very careful with sweet fizzy drinks, fruit juice drinks, yogurt drinks, and squash drinks. Typically, these beverages are loaded with processed sugar.

I did consume a considerable amount in my youth when I ate unmindfully. Clearly the extra weight I carried at that time, was closely related to the consumption of these drinks and the overly processed foods, that were prevalent in my meals/snacks. I am no longer keen on these beverages. I am very thankful that I am no longer one of many who seem to need a can or more of Coke or other similar type drink(s) every day. Thankfully, we can wean ourselves off processed foods and drinks—I did. It is not easy but doable. In Chapter 11, I discuss a strategy that works better than the method I used many years ago--seeking the Lord's help.

I do not recommend substituting these sugar-laden drinks with low-calorie alternatives. These are discussed below.

The popularity of coffee shops around the world has also increased the consumption of various coffees, lattes, chocolate, and other similar type beverages. These often contain a lot of sugar and cream, and therefore increased saturated fat and calories. They can easily contain a substantial amount or more of one's recommended daily intake of sugar, fat, and calories in one go. Food for thought, right?

I know that sometimes we desire to have a drink other than water that has some flavor to it. There is nothing wrong with that. It is wise though to keep a watchful eye on the amount of sugar contained in what we drink. I will occasionally have a malt drink, usually Amstel Malt, and fresh fruit infused water.

## Diet Foods and Drinks

I am not keen on reduced calorie foods and drinks. They contain sugar substitutes that leave an unpleasant after-taste. If my memory serves me well, many artificially flavored foods and drinks are also often excessively sweet. I found them quite sickening. They are also not nearly as satisfying as the foods and drinks free of these substitutes. For example, a one-inch slice of rich cake is much more satiating than a two-inch slice of reduced calorie/low carb cake. The negative impact of these foods/drinks is discussed later in this chapter.

## Processed Food and Drink Production

According to Michael Moss,[20] giant food corporations have manipulated ingredients to establish the necessary "bliss point" in a very calculating manner. This point is obtained by scientifically determining the precise amount of salt, processed sugar, and unhealthy fats to get consumers hooked. These amounts are frequently copious. Moss describes sugar as having a "high-speed, blunt assault on our brains" and refers to it as the "methamphetamine of processed food ingredients." He sees fat as the opiate: "a smooth operator whose effects are less obvious, but no less powerful." He observes that, without salt, processed food companies would cease to exist.

Food giants really do go to great length to achieve their goals, incurring high research and development costs. All with an endgame of ensuring that the exact formulations of junk foods and drinks get their customers addicted. These foods should be eaten very sparingly, if at all.

It is also important to know that processed foods are designed to make us want more. It is therefore easy to lose control of the amounts eaten with these foods. On the other hand, real foods are wholesome and more filling. For example, it is not uncommon to gulp down a pint-size glass of a sugary fizzy drink. It would be difficult, I dare say uncomfortable, to do the same with a similar quantity of freshly squeezed organic oranges. The former is processed and the latter more wholesome and filling. When we eat/drink real foods/drinks, we consume the right amounts—what our bodies need. Conversely, we often consume excessive quantities of junk foods/drinks.[21]

I recall that with ultra-processed foods I would eat voluminous amounts and feel unsatisfied. It really is no wonder that these foods can cause us to overeat when consumed without checks and discretion. And with the often-excessive amounts of sugar and saturated fat they are well-known for, they add unnecessary calories to our meals. The result here will certainly be weight gain among other unfavorable outcomes. The reverse is the case with real, nutrient- dense foods. They are filling and satisfying with hunger curbing fiber that helps us keep control of the amounts consumed.

### How to Consume Processed Foods and Beverages

Processed foods are mostly consumed as "easy," ready-to-eat meals, as well as snacks and desserts. With the busy lives experienced by many and the increased availability of these foods, people have been eating more of them recently, with a negative impact on waistlines and on overall health. We must not let the fast pace of this world cause us to look solely to the "convenient" solutions provided by these foods.[22] At the cost of sounding like a broken record, I will say it again: *processed foods and drinks should be consumed as sparingly as possible.*

Many will eat a meal comprising of solely processed foods and drinks. This is not at all conducive to good health. I was guilty of this decades ago. I believe one of the easiest ways to keep control of the portion sizes of these overly processed foods is to eat a small portion of the sweet foods as dessert after a good nutritious meal. This is wise, as most store-bought muffins, cupcakes, etc., often pack in a full day's allowance of sugar, in what is sold as a portion. Perhaps the savory items can be an addition to a meal as opposed to being eaten on an empty stomach. We should also not feel compelled to consume full portions; there is nothing wrong with eating only a slice of a muffin, for instance. This will keep a healthy check on the amounts we consume. Remember: moderation is key.

### More Negative Effects of Processed Sugar, Foods, and Drinks

We now know how detrimental processed sugar can be to our general well-being in the short- and long-term. Another worthwhile reminder of the malady that can be caused by drinks and processed foods with a high sugar content is that they have a high GI and can cause our insulin levels to rise. This was discussed in the previous chapter. This is a risk factor for weight gain and obesity. Obesity can also increase our risk of cancer. I discuss the cancer connection later in this chapter.

There are studies that have documented the impact of processed foods/drinks. Fifty to sixty years ago, in countries in Africa and in Australia, when these products were first introduced, research shows that within only 3 months there was an increase in the diagnosis of obesity, cardiovascular disease,[23] fatty liver disease, etc. We ought to be very wary of these foods; they are not at all healthy. They are quite addictive too, apparently more so than cigarettes, alcohol, and cocaine. This means that those addicted to MAD foods would find it more difficult being weaned off these foods than off cigarettes, alcohol, and cocaine.[24] Quite frightening, don't you think?

We should not be surprised if we eat junk and our body experiences all sorts of problems. If we fill our car with adulterated fuel, it will not run at its optimum. Our body is even more complex than a car.[25] The digestion of our food, hormone levels, and our moods are all interconnected.[26]

Did you know that processed foods can cause depression?[27] Charlize Theron, an Oscar-winning actress, purposely put on weight twice for film roles by snacking on processed foods. Her choice was primarily potato chips, of which she ate voluminous amounts. These foods affected Charlize's mood, and she found herself dealing with depression for the first time in her life. She also felt constantly lethargic and tired and found it hard to break the cycle of bad eating. Eventually she did manage to stop eating these highly processed foods but struggled for a time, not feeling good about herself. It really can make one depressed eating large amounts of processed foods over long periods.[28]

I, too, recall frequently feeling tired, lethargic, and somewhat depressed when I ate many of these highly processed foods unmindfully, many years ago. Since I started eating well, I am never lethargic or depressed. If I have slept well the night before and am in good health, I do not feel tired during the day.

It would be wrong of me to not credit the general well-being I enjoy now, and have for a long time, to my relationship with God above all else. My faith in His promises gives me peace and fills me with joy.

Charlize Theron found it easier to lose the weight the first time, as she was younger. In the second film, she put on as much as 50 pounds. This was more weight than the first time, and she found it more difficult to shed. We will do ourselves well if we learn to eat healthy early, as it does get harder to lose weight as we age. I discussed the benefits of learning to eat well as a child in the previous chapter.

My brother recently cut back on processed foods and drinks. He lost about 20 pounds in less than 5 months without doing much else. What does this tell you? It tells me that processed foods and drinks, should be consumed very sparingly, if at all. They often contain a ton of sugar and other ingredients; we will do our bodies well to avoid them.

Many studies correlate that consuming excessive processed sugar has an adverse effect on our bodies and can increase the risk of cancer. In researching for this book, I had the opportunity of discussing the impact of this sugar on our bodies with a cancer specialist. There is a consensus that excessive amounts of processed sugar in our diet can be detrimental to our health, including increasing the risk of cancer.[29]

Consuming excessive amounts of these products will certainly mean more calories that can cause weight gain and increased body fat and obesity in extreme cases. Obesity does not cause cancer, but it can increase the chances of developing cancer. Typically, there will be other underlying conditions present for this to be the case. These could include someone who is overweight, who might have a genetic predisposition to cancer, and who drinks alcohol and/or sugary beverages, and smokes.

In the case of obese women, fat tissue can increase oestrogen levels that may increase the risk for those predisposed to oestrogen-related breast cancer. Oestrogen feeds these cancers. The broken-down sugar from consumed processed foods/drinks can feed tumors in untreated cancers which cause them to thrive. The verdict is out: there *is* some correlation between our lifestyle and cancer.

Processed sugar and foods also negatively affect arthritis. People who are arthiritic, and eat excessive amounts of processed sugar, can cause their bodies to release cytokines. These are pro-inflammatory proteins. The inflammation will cause pain, swelling and joint stiffness—yet another reason to be cautious of theses sugars.[30]

It is also interesting to note that the effects of these highly processed sweet items on the aging process can be quite "bitter." According to Rebecca Adams in a HuffPost Style and Beauty Article, Updated December 7, 2017, sugar is as bad for our skin as it is for our waistline; when we ingest processed sugars, or high glycemic foods that cause our glucose levels to spike, our insulin levels rise. According to Dr. Nicholas Perricone, a dermatologist and nutritionist, this leads to what he describes as "a burst of inflammation throughout the body." Inflammation causes enzymes to be produced that break down collagen and elastin. This results in sagging skin and wrinkles.

Digested sugar attaches to the collagen in our skin through a process called glycation. In addition to aging, glycation can exacerbate skin conditions like acne. I recall having quite a few pimples many years ago when I ate unmindfully. My skin breakouts were often aggravated after I indulged in highly processed sweet foods. My skin has been pimple free for the most part over the last 25+ years. I had no idea about this and other adverse effects of processed sugars on our bodies, until I researched as I wrote this book.

This is yet another reason to avoid various store-baked goods with copious amounts of added refined sugar, as this may help keep wrinkles at bay. If you cannot stop eating sweets and sugar-laden biscuits until the packet is finished, *do not buy them*. They are meant to be treats not meals.

Very briefly, another downside to processed sugar is that it affects the pH balance of our bodies, which thrive better when they are more alkaline. Processed sugar makes us more acidic. Acidity provides a favorable environment for disease, and it increases our risk for numerous problems including chronic inflammation and kidney stones. Over time inflammation may lead to several health problems such as heart disease, diabetes, liver disease, and cancer.[31]

Conversely natural sugars have not been linked to inflammation. Typically, many natural foods containing natural sugars, such as veggies and fruits, are anti-inflammatory.[32]

Many people think that it is alright to replace processed sugar with the various substitutes available. It is not. Often people try to curb their sweet cravings by grabbing a diet soda, with its promise of reduced calories. Unfortunately, this choice may actually sabotage this intention, the reason being that artificial sweeteners might fool our taste buds, but our brain and digestive system know the difference and will therefore ramp up their efforts to obtain the real thing. This can cause the consumption of way more calories. I can totally relate to this. It was my experience many years ago...

Several large studies dating back as far as the 1970s have found that the sustained intake of artificial sweeteners, like aspartame and sucralose, actually can lead to increased weight.

This is so as tasting sweet flavors tends to increase our desire and dependence on sweet foods. Therefore, artificial sweeteners can indeed make us crave more sweet things. Over time, the increased appetite and sweet cravings can lead to eating more and gaining weight. This is not what most people would expect from consuming reduced calorie products.[33] Artificial sweeteners may also alter gut bacteria.[34] The impotence of a healthy gut on our well-being is discussed in Chapter 10.

According to a new study by the American Heart Association and American Stroke Association,[35] drinking a couple of any kind of artificially sweetened drinks per day was linked to an increased risk of clot-based strokes, heart attacks, and early death in women over 50. The risks were found to be higher for obese and/or black American women with no history of heart disease or diabetes. Previous research also showed a link between artificially sweetened diet beverages and stroke, dementia, type 2 diabetes, obesity, and metabolic syndrome, which can lead to heart disease and diabetes.

The study by the American Heart and American Stroke Association is confirmation that there is a relationship between artificially sweetened beverages and vascular risks. The results do not show causation, but the findings are enough reason to cause us to pay attention according to the American Academy of Neurology President Dr. Ralph Sacco. Apparently, more studies are necessary to determine what, in these sweeteners, causes these maladies.

According to **Mossavar-Rahmani**, black American women without a previous history of heart or diabetes are about four times more likely to have a clot-based stroke. In white women, the risks are different. They are 1.3 times more likely to have coronary heart disease. According to North Carolina cardiologist Dr. Kevin Campbell, "post-menopausal women tend to have a higher risk for vascular disease because they are lacking the protective effects of natural hormones." This could contribute to an increased risk of stroke and heart disease.

In my opinion, this is evidence to make us cautious about consuming excessive amounts of artificially sweetened foods/beverages. It certainly has made me wonder about these reduced calorie foods/drinks I am so thankful that the unpleasant taste I experienced many years ago kept me away from all these products. I am told that their tastes have since improved. There is no going back for me though. We really will do ourselves a world of good to drink more water and other natural beverages like fresh fruit infused water and unsweetened herbal teas. I promise you when you make a conscious decision to start eating/drinking and enjoying real foods/drinks, and you see the benefits, it is unlikely you will return to an unhealthy way of eating.

While writing this book, I had discussions with a few people, some of whom were strangers, who appeared to have their weight under control. They all unanimously had the viewpoint that processed sugars were to be consumed cautiously, very sparingly.

I must include in this chapter, even if very briefly, the fact that we ingest sugar from many other carb-rich foods. Some of these are processed but healthy. Foods like whole wheat pasta, brown rice, whole grain bread and other healthy carb-rich foods also break down into sugar upon ingestion. That is why it is possible to have a high blood sugar level, even when we avoid foods and drinks containing overly processed sugars.

We need to keep an eye on carb rich foods, more so if we are diabetic or have a predisposition. There are many healthy carb rich foods, such as brown rice, mangoes, and pineapples. These and others were discussed extensively in Chapter 3. That said, healthy carbs are a better, more wholesome source of sugar than the refined variety obtained from processed foods. They often also contain fiber and other nutrients. Again, with all foods, moderation is key. Our intention with all processed foods and drinks should be an awareness of the quantities and frequency with which we consume them.

I have to say, that after my extensive research and findings in writing this book, I have found myself shying away even more from these food products. I will say no more, except to remind us that we are all here with a distinct, unique purpose. We should endeavor to feed our bodies-- God's temple--with healthy foods. A reminder here of this scripture is worthwhile:

**1 Corinthians 3:16 KJV**
*Know ye not that ye are the temple of God, and that the Spirit of God dwelleth in you?*

We must strive always to keep our bodies well. It is a major step in helping us fulfill His purpose and His perfect will for our lives.

# Chapter 6

# Fasting

Fasting is a planned abstinence from food, drink, or both for a specified time. It can also be absolute or dry—the abstinence from all foods and liquids for a predetermined period. I will not dwell on this latter fast.

Fasting can be embarked on for spiritual reasons. It is also a good way to reset our eating habits after being off track, for instance after a vacation or a period of indulgence such as at Christmas and Thanksgiving.

Have you ever wondered why your eating habits often change while you are on vacation? It is because social norms in a particular environment can affect eating behavior without your awareness; so, your eating can be influenced by where you are.[1] This deviation can cause weight gain. Fasting is a useful way to gradually return to previous eating habits when you return home.

Fasting can also be useful to jumpstart a weight loss regime. There are various fasts. Many claim that they can help with weight loss and cleansing. Let's look at a few.

### The Daniel Fast[2]

The Daniel Fast is a religious partial fast. It is named after Daniel in the Bible who decided not to eat food from King Nebuchadnezzar, as he was associated with idol worship. He first embarked on a 10 day fast and increased it to 21 days after his well-being proved that his health was not in any way impaired by the fast. Proponents of this fast claim that it produces both physical and spiritual breakthroughs. So, whether it is a health condition, emotional concerns, or spiritual bondage, the Daniel Fast can help us experience a breakthrough.

## Step 1

This fast typically lasts for 10-21 days. During this time, meat, wine, gluten, and other rich foods should be avoided in favor of nutrient dense vegetables, fruits, nuts, seeds, and whole grains (gluten-free only). It is recommended that one's water intake be increased too; this is always a good idea.

This fast is like a vegan diet as it excludes animal products. The Daniel Fast also excludes white flour, all processed foods, sweeteners, preservatives, additives, and caffeine. Apparently, the first three days are often tough, but it gets easier. A general feeling of well-being and an accompanying glow are additional expected benefits from this fast.

## Step 2

Spending scheduled prayer times with God every day.

## Step 3

With this fast, Daniel proved to the king that he could do his job more efficiently. The fast also helped him increase in wisdom and knowledge, as he spent quality time with God. Proponents of this fast advise us to imitate Daniel during this fast by praying, working on our skills, setting goals, and pursuing excellence. These are worthwhile traits to work on always.

I have not done the Daniel Fast but, in my opinion, anything that draws us closer to God can only be good. I also think that its duration is not prohibitive, so one is unlikely to have crippling cravings for foods forfeited while on this fast. It is also a great jumpstart to healthy living, as it is likely to help us desire healthy foods. These will help us in our quest to eat intentionally and fuel our body, His temple, respectfully.

## Juice and Vegetable Fasting

Juice fasting, also known as juice cleansing and juicing, is a diet in which only fruit and vegetable juices are consumed while abstaining from solid foods.[3] Proponents of this fast have made claims that it can help with detoxification and help curb sugar cravings. It typically lasts for 2-7 days and involves the blending of a few fruits and/or vegetables, sometimes with spices. Cayenne pepper is a popular spice used in these fasts. It detoxifies, stimulates circulation, neutralizes acidity, and aids digestion.

Some dieticians and doctors are not convinced of the benefits of prolonged juiced vegetables and fruits on the body. Regarding the detoxifying properties of juicing, it is believed that our body is designed to eliminate wastes and toxins on its own. Another concern is the elimination of pulp and therefore fiber in the preparation of these juices.[4] Another criticism of juicing is that, depending on the type and its duration, these so-called detox diets can have far-reaching consequences. These may include muscle loss and an unhealthy regaining of weight lost plus extra added weight. This can happen, as it is not uncommon for food bingeing to follow these fasts. Our bodies tend to crave foods that they were deprived of during the fast. In addition, juice mixes containing grapefruit juice may adversely interact with some prescription drugs.[5]

I personally have never embarked on a total juicing fast. I once went on a cleansing fast, which included fresh juices, protein shakes, a variety of lightly steamed vegetables, and some vitamins. It lasted 10 days. I did lose weight and my skin had an amazing glow. I craved many foods that were prohibited during the fast as soon as it was over. These included meat, fish, grains, and legumes. I very quickly put back all the lost weight, but thankfully nothing extra. I honestly believe the only reason I did not put on any additional weight was because I was already disciplined with food before the fast and quickly returned to my moderate way of eating.

### Intermittent Fasting[6]

This is currently one of the world's most popular trends in health and fitness. It is a pattern of eating and abstaining, alternating when food is consumed and not (fasting). The fasting period typically lasts for at least 12 hours, when only water should be consumed. No tea, herbal or not, coffee, diet soda, chewing gum, vitamins, or mints should be ingested during the fasting period. Basically, this means nothing that could cause the body to have a digestive response. There are 24 hours in a day; so, if one eats for 12 hours and fasts for 12 hours, they are on a 12-12 plan.

In embarking on this fast, we should pick the time that suits us. Many proponents recommend starting the fasting period after our last food or drink consumption before bedtime. Overtime, we could work on increasing the fasting period to up to 13-14 hours, if possible. In my study, I encountered 16-8 and even 20-4 plan—the former numbers being the fasting period and the latter the period when food is consumed. I personally believe that the 16-8 and 20-4 plans would be tough. Currently, popular intermittent fasts involve 16-8 and 14-10 plans, and are typically done a couple of times per week.

The emphasis in intermittent fasting is not really on the foods consumed, but rather on when they are eaten. It is more an eating pattern than a diet plan.

It is recommended that these fasts be broken with a no-calorie drink like green tea other teas or coffee, followed by a nutrient dense meal, which can include greens, good carbs, good proteins, and good fats. This could be a green smoothie with avocado or sugar-free peanut butter added, or green vegetables cooked with garlic and olive oil and served with some protein such as eggs, and/or fish. During this fast, as always, it is beneficial to drink plenty of water. It not only helps food move along in our digestive systems, it keeps us full and curtails food cravings.

The benefits of this type of fasting include weight loss and improved overall health. Decreased insulin levels can be experienced during this fast, which helps us burn excess body fat. Proponents of intermittent fasting suggest that another benefit is that it gives our bodies a break from constantly digesting food. In this time, the body is then able to better perform any repairs needed. These benefits are different for everyone.

I found researching this type of fasting very interesting, as it pretty much sums up the way I eat regularly. This has been my practice for nearly 30 years. I typically finish eating my last meal for the day before 7 p.m. and will have nothing thereafter but water until about 9-10 a.m. the following morning when I have breakfast. I am therefore generally on a 14-10 plan. I fast for 14 hours and eat during a 10-hour period. It is worthwhile noting that I am not famished by the time I have my breakfast, except when I have exercised.

I wondered if this manner of eating contributed to maintaining my weight over more than 25 years. Perhaps if I ate unmindfully or binged during my eating periods, I would have experienced very different results.

In my opinion, these fasts are not a harmful addition to our lifestyle. The juicing and Daniel fasts can also play some role in jumpstarting a weight loss program and/or getting back on track after we have indulged in excess eating for whatever reason. The Daniel Fast also enhances our spiritual well-being.

Fasts should not be followed with excessive amounts of food. It is best to reintroduce food carefully, spacing out meals in smaller portions.

Today, many do not remember me when I was over-weight, or "chubby," as I saw myself years ago. Others do not believe I could have been any different than the way I have been for over 25 years.

They say a picture is worth a thousand words...

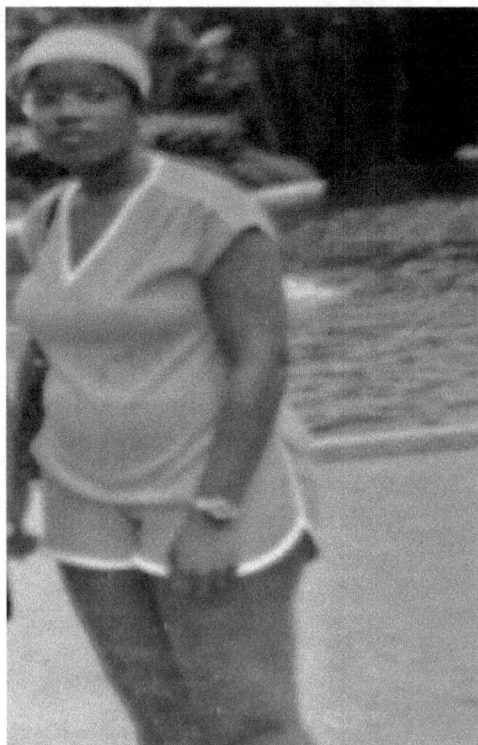

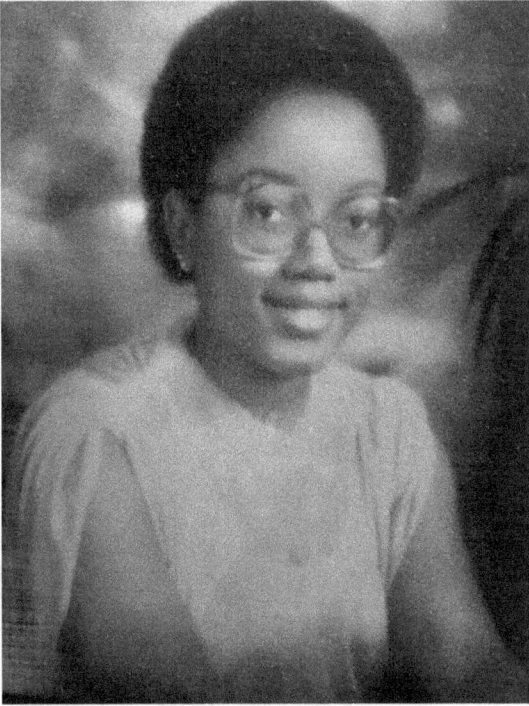

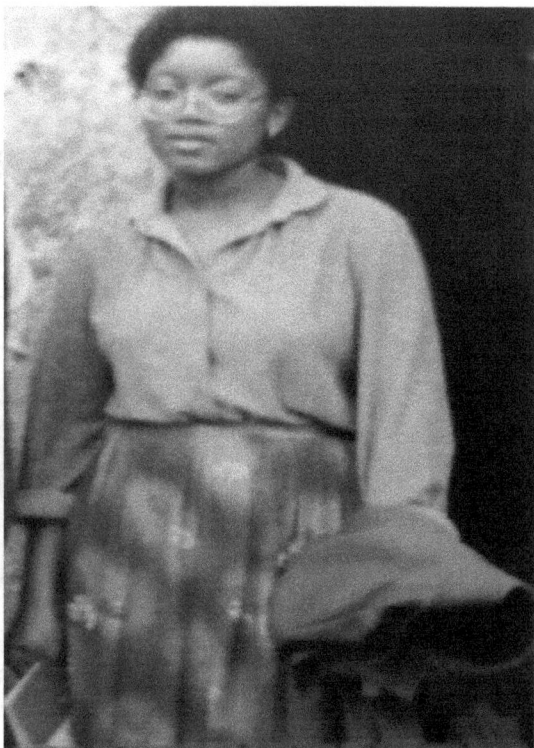

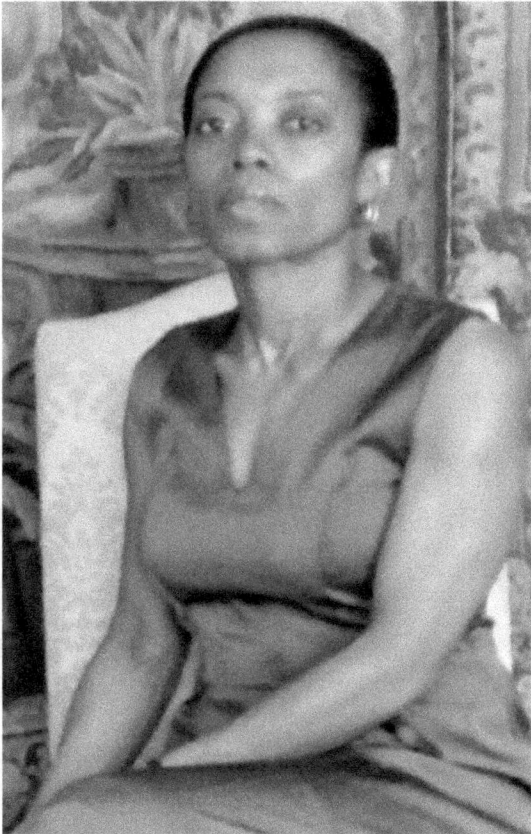

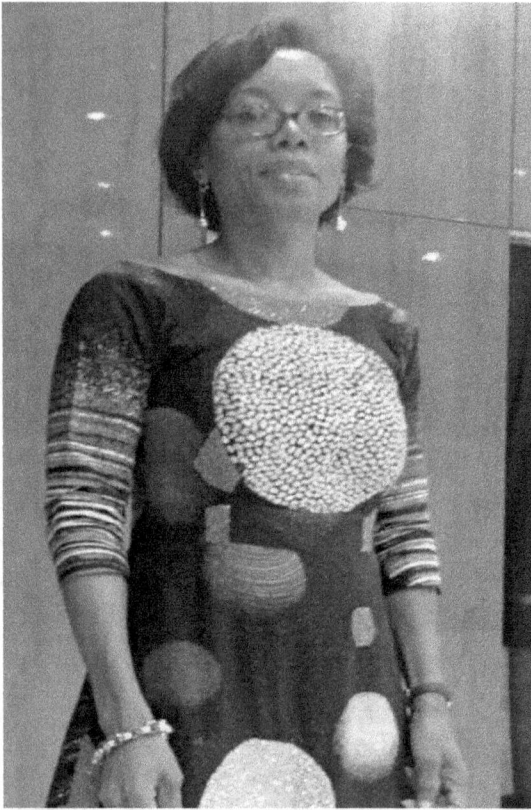

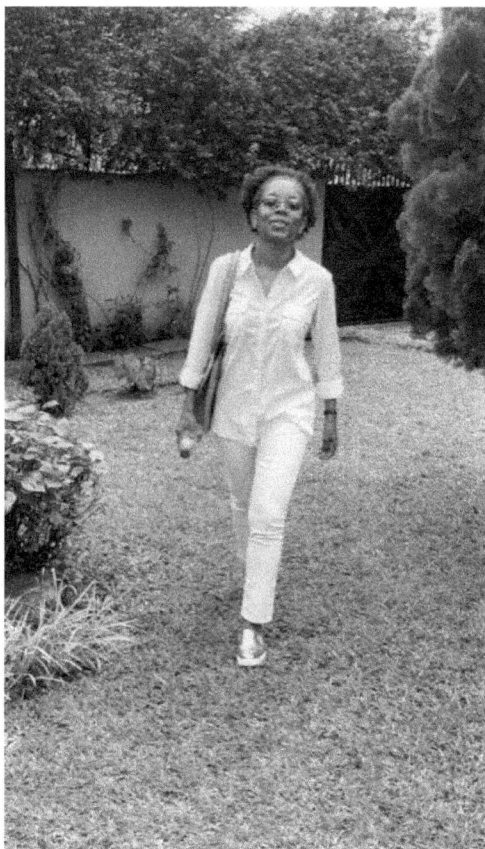

# Chapter 7

# Metabolism

Metabolism is a highly misunderstood topic. I have learned more about metabolism in my research and have had to debunk some ideas, which I now understand obscure the truth.[1]

Metabolism is the whole range of biochemical processes that occur within living organisms and is a necessary part of life. It generally refers to the breakdown of food and its conversion into energy.

Our resting metabolism (basal metabolic rate) measures how many calories we burn while we are doing nothing. It accounts for a huge amount of the total calories we burn each day. The foods we fuel our body with provide all the energy we require.

According to Alexxai Kravitz, a neuroscientist and obesity researcher at the National Institutes of Health, our basal metabolic rate accounts for 60% to 80% of total energy expenditure. Surprisingly, physical activity accounts for a comparatively minuscule part of our total energy expenditure, only about 10-30% of total energy output. This increases considerably if one is a professional athlete, has a very physically demanding job, or exerts a lot of energy otherwise. The digestion of our food accounts for about 10% of total energy expenditure.

Even though exercise results in relatively small amounts of total energy expenditure, it is invaluable in combination with good nutrition that includes significant amounts of protein for increasing our lean muscle ratio. This affects our metabolism. Exercise is discussed a little further below and more extensively in the next chapter.

Metabolism can vary widely among people, but researchers do not really understand why. Two people with similar size and body composition can have very different metabolic rates. The reasons for this are not fully understood. According to Will Wong, a researcher and professor at the Johns Hopkins Center for Metabolism and Obesity Research, "We don't understand the mechanism that controls a person's metabolism."

Generally, there are predictors of how fast a person's metabolism will work. These include the amount of lean muscle and fat tissue in an individual's body, genetics, age, and sex. At any given weight, the leaner we are the less fat we have, the higher will be our metabolic rate. This is because muscle uses a lot more energy than fat while at rest. Many have thought pills, exercise, etc., can manipulate metabolism. It really is not as simple as that. Only exercise, which increases lean muscle, will eventually have an impact on metabolism. Genetics influence our metabolism. However, the verdict is not yet out as to why some families have higher or lower metabolic rates.

Our metabolism slows down as we age. Therefore, an individual who manages to retain roughly the same amount of fat and muscle tissue over a long period may still find a slowdown in their metabolism. This is likely to manifest in someone having to reduce their food intake in order to maintain their weight. An increase in weight as we age is perhaps also related to decreased activity.

Women with comparable statistics to men, tend to burn fewer calories. Some women have a higher metabolic rate during the second half of their menstrual cycle. This is referred to as the Luteal Phase. This is the period between ovulation and menstruation. It typically lasts for 14 days with the resting metabolic rate increasing by up to 10%.

The way we fuel our bodies also has an impact on our metabolism. Our eating plans, when trying to lose or maintain our weight, must never come at the expense of good nutrition. We should always focus on eating whole, nutritious foods that nourish our bodies avoiding overly processed sugars and diet foods. In fact, we should treat them as *poison*.

Apparently, it is a myth that small portions of food spread out through the day help boost metabolism. More important is our body's muscle mass. We will therefore do well to increase the amount of lean muscle and reduce the fat tissue in our bodies. The best way is by eating moderate amounts of healthy foods (increasing our protein intake will be beneficial here. This is discussed later in this chapter) in combination with exercise. Typically, when we gain fat, we lose muscle and vice versa.

Generally speaking, months or years of dieting (especially greatly reduced calorie food plans over a long period) may result in poor nutrition and is likely to lead to muscle loss, which we now know slows down metabolism. This ultimately results in our bodies burning fewer calories with possible weight gain.

It is not easy to speed up our metabolism. However, we can do things to our body to slow it down. Here are some strategies for losing fat and keeping it off and building muscle, which will help ensure that we do not cause our metabolism to slowdown.

**Water[2]**

Our body requires water in all its cells, tissues, and organs to help regulate its temperature and maintain other bodily functions. Water is essential for the digestion of our food. Remember that the foods we eat provide 100% of our energy requirements. Our basal metabolic rate accounts for 60% to 80% of this. Even mild dehydration can slow down this rate and our metabolism. In a study published in The Journal of Clinical Endocrinology and Metabolism, researchers found water to have an effect on metabolism. To stay hydrated, we should drink eight or more glasses of water daily. We should strive to make water our drink of choice. It is the elixir of life.

## Protein[3]

Protein is found throughout the body, in every tissue, and particularly in our muscles. Consuming protein is essential when trying to lose fat and helps develop and keep that all-important lean body mass. We need to consume more protein in tandem with exercise and weightlifting in order to achieve increased muscle mass.

Other benefits of protein are that it increases satiety and helps us feel full with less food. In addition, our body burns more calories when digesting protein than it does digesting carbohydrates or fats. We can try replacing some carbs with lean protein and weightlifting to increase our muscle mass and so boost our metabolism. Turkey, chicken, fish, nuts, eggs, and beans, are all good sources of protein.

## Green Tea[4]

This tea contains caffeine, which has been found to elevate metabolism for a couple of hours. Not everyone experiences this with green tea, though. I do, and so generally avoid it as it makes me lose weight. I did drink it often, when I needed to lose weight over 25 years ago. I now find it useful when I want to indulge. For instance, if I indulge in a calorie-laden dessert or have been eating more than usual, such as over Christmas or while on vacation, I will drink a couple of cups of green tea. More often than not, my weight will remain stable.

Many people are sensitive to caffeine and find that their sleep is disrupted after ingesting it. If this applies to you, I suggest you try the decaf varieties that are now available.

Sleep is a very important factor in weight loss and weight management. The impact of sleep to our well-being is discussed further in Chapter 10.

## Black Coffee[5]

Taken in moderation coffee can cause a rise in metabolism in the short-term. It can also increase endurance during exercise and is a good pick-me-up when tired. Anyone whose sleep is disrupted by caffeine should be careful. Perhaps only try consuming it early and avoid it later in the day.

## Spices[6]

Spicy foods contain natural chemicals that increase metabolism. To enjoy these benefits, add chili peppers to food when cooking. These benefits are probably only temporary and miniscule but, if spicy foods are eaten often enough, the benefits may add up.

## Crash Diets

Crash diets usually involve greatly reduced food consumption and other restrictions, such as none or very limited carbs. These diets often slow our metabolic rate by slowing down our resting metabolism. As we now know, our basal metabolic rate accounts for a significant percentage (over 50%) of total energy expenditure. According to The Mayo Clinic's Michael Jensen, with slow, gradual weight loss, our metabolic rate holds out well.[7] This is another reason why a slow and steady weight loss program ensures the best results.

We should always say no to crash diets. They may initially result in weight loss but usually at a cost--the expense of good nutrition. As discussed earlier, they may also lead to muscle loss with resulting reduction in metabolism.

When this happens, the body starts to burn fewer calories. Oftentimes extra weight is also gained.

Another common scenario with crash dieting involves eating very little for long periods and not experiencing the desired results. Some people can even gain weight, because they have probably lost muscle mass and so burn fewer calories. Not eating well and starving ourselves generally causes a decrease in our lean muscle to fat ratio and subsequently to our metabolism.

The ideal plan is to eat nutrient-dense foods in moderation in conjunction with a balanced exercise regime. This will likely help ensure that our metabolism is at its optimal level.

### Exercise

Our bodies are constantly burning calories, even when we are inactive. This resting metabolic rate is higher in individuals with a higher muscle than fat ratio. A good exercise routine combined with wholesome nutrition is the ultimate way to increase lean muscle mass. The role of exercise in weight loss, weight maintenance, and in increased metabolism is discussed in more detail in the next chapter.

### Hormones[8]

The hormones that the thyroid gland produces control the speed of an individual's metabolism. This is discussed in more detail in Chapter 10.

### Conclusion

We should strive to ensure that we do not cause our metabolism to slow down. The best way is by increasing and maintaining our body's muscle mass and reducing our fat tissue. This will result in a leaner looking body. With a lean body, we attain a higher resting metabolism, which will assist us with quickly burning the fuel with which we feed our bodies.

# Chapter 8

# Physical Activity and Exercise

We have looked at the role of diet in our quest for a healthy lifestyle. Now let's look at exercise. A healthy lifestyle is part exercise but mainly good nutrition—a ratio of 20% exercise and 80% nutrition. We cannot eat uncontrollably and think that some activity in the mix is enough to maintain or lose weight. Just as with food, striking a good balance with exercise is beneficial.

Let's take a look at physical activity and exercise. They are both important components of a healthy lifestyle. These terms are often misused or used interchangeably. Physical activity requires energy and involves movement that is carried out by our muscles. Any movement one does is physical activity.[1]

The World Health Organization (WHO) has identified physical inactivity[2] (a predominantly sedentary lifestyle and/or a lack of exercise) as an independent risk factor for chronic disease development. It is now the fourth leading cause of death worldwide.

On the other hand, exercise is defined as planned, structured, repetitive, and intentional physical effort embarked on with the aim of sustaining or improving health and maintaining our fitness levels. Research shows that all physical activity has a positive impact on our health and wellness. Exercise improves cardiovascular health, endurance, strength, flexibility, and body composition.[3]

It has been suggested that we need at least 150 minutes of moderate aerobic activity or 75 minutes of vigorous aerobic activity a week or a combination of these to maintain a healthy lifestyle.[4] Aerobic activity involves cardiovascular conditioning, with our breathing and heart rate increased for a sustained period of time.[5] However, it is not good to be mostly sedentary as we commute, work at our desk, and generally be a couch potato for the greater part of our day. High levels of inactivity through the day can very quickly nullify the little exercise done and cause major health problems.

We should all strive to become more physically active by standing more often than sitting during and after work. We should walk and use stairs instead of elevators whenever possible. Safety is important always though, so if stairs are isolated it is probably safer to use elevators. We should endeavor to develop a habit of taking walks during our lunch break. In safe parking lots we should park some distance away from the entrance and walk. At home we can increase our physical activity by gardening or doing various exercises with weights while we watch television.

Let us compare French and American physical activity habits.[6] The French are not super sporty like Americans or others with various exercises, like running marathons, weightlifting, attending gym classes, etc. They are, however, consistently more active. They walk a lot to work, to pick up their children, and through the Metro. This is particularly so for Parisians. There are virtually no escalators in France, and so they readily climb stairs. They incorporate moderate physical activity every day, mastering the art of keeping physically active without really trying. The result is that the rate of obesity in France is about a third of that in the US. The French also typically eat less than Americans do. This was discussed in Chapter 4.

I will now concentrate on exercise as planned physical activity. I have known people who exercise quite well and regularly but do not enjoy the desired results. This is very often because of bad eating habits. As I mentioned earlier, it is futile to eat uncontrollably and think that some activity in the mix is enough. My experience has always been that when I am eating well (clean eating), my body responds better and quicker to exercise. It really is phenomenal; try it and see for yourself.

Exercise is essential to help us feel and look our best. The kind of exercise we choose will ultimately be driven by what we enjoy and feel comfortable doing and our goals. Exercise is also a great stress buster. Our goals should be set to get us healthy and fit. This does not necessarily equate to being skinny, as our bodies are all built differently.

We should not waste time dwelling on the difficulty of changing our bad habits, such as a previously sedentary lifestyle. Rather we should focus our attention on the results and all the ways being healthy will transform our lives for the better.[7] Exercise will make us healthier. It is also exhilarating as it releases the "feel good" and "happy" hormone: endorphins.[8] They are responsible for the satisfied feeling we get after a completed workout, the joyful anticipation of the next session, or just the growing confidence in our own capabilities.

With exercise, small steps are powerful and life-changing, particularly if we have previously been sedentary. Intentional small, incremental steps in our exercise routine are vital to transitioning from an unhealthy lifestyle to a healthy one; they are vital to stepping into the fullness of our new selves.[9]

There are so many different forms of exercise to choose from: walking, jogging, running, swimming, weightlifting, kickboxing, shadowboxing, spinning, aerobic classes, etc. We should pick the forms of exercise we think we will enjoy. I recommend doing a variety. This will keep our bodies responding (see explanation in next paragraph), and keep it exciting, too.

It is imperative that we do not stick to the same routine for too long. We need to mix it up so that our bodies keep responding. I like to see it as shocking our body to keep it from knowing exactly what to expect. We should strive to keep our bodies guessing. We get the best results that way. If we do not mix it up, our efforts can start to be of no effect. When this happens, we can go to the gym for years and remain the same. This is very discouraging and can cause us to give up. We must learn to exercise smartly and avoid the complacency that can easily set in.

I have seen many people at the gym who attend religiously but have absolutely nothing to show for it. This could be for a number of reasons. They are doing the same routine day in and day out, and their bodies have stopped reacting or their eating is outrunning their exercise regimen. These are the most common reasons for non-productive exercise routines. It is a waste of our time to continue doing the same thing when the desired results are not being attained. Getting on a varied moderate exercise and healthy eating plan should give us worthwhile results.

If you have not exercised in a long time, or ever, walking is a good start. Begin with a slow to moderate pace for at least 30 minutes, say three times in the first week. Try to increase to five times by the third or fourth week. At that point, increase your pace to a brisk walk and start to use your arms to propel yourself forward. This is referred to as "power walking." It is also beneficial to hold light dumbbells for added resistance.

You can then progress slowly to a mix of walking and a gentle jog for a week or two. Then try gentle jogging for up to 30 minutes for 3 times per week, if you can. When this gets comfortable, you should try increasing your pace to a run. You should work on increasing your distance and mixing your jog with short and fast sprints. This is another good variation. Remember to wear good walking and/or running shoes and replace them when worn-out to keep your feet, ankles, and knees healthy.

Swimming is another good form of exercise. Mixing it up in the pool is essential, too. You can do this with different strokes—breaststroke, backstroke, butterfly stroke, etc. Also, doing water aerobics every now and again is beneficial and fun. The resistance the water gives makes it fun and exhilarating.

I particularly enjoy weightlifting and now concentrate more on this form of exercise than on others. I do different routines mixed with a little cardio and like the definition that it has given my body. With more muscles, metabolism is also increased, as we discussed in the previous Chapter.

It is worthwhile paying a personal trainer to help you learn how to use the different equipment in the gym. It is very important to learn how to use them properly for good form, to avoid and/or minimize injury, and to get the desired results. Never settle for asking other gym users how to use the equipment. Trust me, there are very few things that are more irritating than a gym novice interrupting the routine of a regular gym attendee to find out how equipment works. Even worse is a novice trying to join a hard-core gym user's routine. This not only interrupts someone's rhythm, it can also lead to injury due to a lapse in concentration.

Many women say they do not want to be muscular. There is typically more fat on the female body than on the male body. Ladies, let me assure you that you would have to work through all your fat to be muscular. That takes super discipline for most women and oftentimes the use of steroids. I am talking about being toned and not flabby, developing enough muscle definition to not only boost metabolism but also to look better in our clothes. In my opinion, it is very attractive to see a woman with a nicely toned butt in jeans and other fitted clothes, and nicely toned arms in sleeveless and short-sleeved dresses and tops.

85

As discussed in the previous chapter, increased muscle mass also helps us have a higher basal metabolic rate. The higher this rate is, the more calories we burn while we are resting.

I have always said that I will never have cosmetic surgery to look better. Whatever I cannot alter with exercise and good eating, I will live with. It is amazing what can be achieved with a good balance in nutrition and exercise-- quantum leaps can be made towards a healthy lifestyle and a leaner body. Try it and see. I honestly think that medical procedures should only be used to save lives. Of course, this is entirely my opinion.

Three women in the public arena who I think have amazing physiques are Gabrielle Union, Jada Pinkett-Smith, and Jennifer Lopez. All three exercise and enjoy their food, too. Jennifer and Jada have proved that having children is no reason to get out of shape. They both have two children and Jennifer carried twins. Jada's mum also looks incredible; she is in her 60s. And no, it's not entirely their genes. They have all mastered the art of mindfully eating and exercising and so are fit and look good. I dare say that if they ate erratically for sustained periods, they would put on weight and certainly be and look less fit. Indeed, I have heard Gabrielle talk about getting back on track after indulging while on vacation.

Now let's look at food intake before and after exercise.[10] Invariably the length and intensity of our planned routine will determine what we should eat and drink. For example, we will require more energy from food to run a marathon than to walk a few miles. To some extent, it is also a matter of preference. Let's pay attention to how we feel during our workout, and let our experience guide us on which pre- and post-exercise eating habits work best for us.

Often, I will not eat before exercising if it is first thing in the morning and it is a short routine. On the other hand, when I exercise later in the day and intensely, I will eat prior to my routine. When I perform intense exercise routines on an empty stomach, I often find that I have less stamina and sometimes even feel lightheaded. There are different views as to whether or not exercising on an empty stomach aids weight loss.[11] In my opinion, it is not a good idea to exercise intensely on a hungry stomach. As I have said, the intensity of exercise is likely to be reduced as one lacks energy.

The foods I tend to consume are typically slow-digesting carbs, protein, and low-fat that are eaten a couple of hours before exercise. I find that these help me work out for a longer duration and/or higher intensity. Carbohydrates supply our body with the glycogen it needs and protein aids in the repairs to any torn muscles. Good and quick pre-workout food options, especially at breakfast, include:

- Whole-grain cereals with almond or other nut "milks" or bread with almond butter (unsweetened)
- Freshly squeezed juice
- A banana
- Yogurt with or without fruit
- An apple with unsweetened peanut or almond butter
- Fruit or protein smoothie
- A bowl of oatmeal with or without fruit

These are my usual choices, there are many more to choose from. We should be careful not to overdo it when it comes to how much we eat before exercise. Eating too much before we exercise can leave us feeling sluggish and even nauseous. This has certainly been my experience. On the other hand, eating too little might not give us the energy required to keep us feeling energized throughout our workout. I find it is best when I eat a meal, at least 90 minutes before I work out, so I do not feel bloated, or a snack 30 minutes before. The key is being aware of how we feel; and doing what works best for us.

If we have not eaten a meal before exercise, it is even more imperative that we eat one after and as soon as possible. These should be protein and carb choices which can help our body recuperate after exercise. When we workout, especially if it involves weight training, we sometimes break down muscle, and there are often small micro tears. Our bodies require food with protein in it to trigger the repair process.[12]

Examples of foods to eat after a workout:

- Lean protein - chicken, fish

- Whole wheat bread with hummus

- Plain Greek yogurt with walnuts and honey

- A couple of boiled eggs with toast

We must remember also that sweating during exercise means that we have lost water as well as electrolytes. When we do not replenish these, we can start to feel dehydrated. This can leave us feeling tired and faint, so bring water to the rescue.

Apparently, failing to eat after exercise can have other repercussions. When we exert ourselves physically our glucose levels will drop. Glucose is essential for brain function as well as our overall energy levels. Low brain function can influence our mood and alertness. Keeping a close watch on glucose levels is particularly important for diabetics.[13] To make the most of our post-workout high, we need to replenish our glucose levels with a well-balanced meal. Let's learn to maximize our workouts by knowing what and when to eat.

We cannot rely on anyone to make our healthy life choices, not our spouses, doctors, or trainers. All they can do is offer support and advice. Ultimately, each of us must take responsibility to eat healthy and exercise. Let's get motivated and choose to be healthy, so that we are better able to fulfill His unique purpose for us. I must emphasize that we cannot accomplish all that we are meant to if our wellbeing is compromised with ill health.

We have to adopt a conscious, purposed approach with exercise as we do with what we eat. When we do not, it is possible to exercise for months and even years without tangible results. Exercise is a beautiful phenomenon. The feel-good hormones released are exhilarating. Do not let those feelings that cause procrastination stop you. Never leave for tomorrow what you can do today. In addition, ignore thoughts that try to tell you the weather is bad. You can exercise indoors. Exercise delivers oxygen and nutrients to our tissues and helps our cardiovascular system work more efficiently.[14] When our heart and lung health improve, we have more energy to tackle daily chores, including fulfilling our purpose.

How we look after our body is entirely our responsibility. What we eat, how we exercise, how we deal with stress, how much rest we get, will all influence our body. We ought therefore to keep a very close watch on these aspects of our lives.

We do not want to push ourselves too hard as to cause injury. The key is moderate exercise. We need to choose routines that we enjoy and keep our bodies fit to help us fulfill God's purpose for our lives.

The Nike saying "Just do it" really motivates me. We can do this, and moderation is key here, too.

# Chapter 9

# Adverse Reactions to Foods

As we make changes to improve our general well-being by eating right, we should also learn to be aware of foods that make us unwell and those that cause adverse reactions. These reactions can be classified as food allergies or intolerance to foods.

Some of these adverse reactions can hinder us and cause discomfort that can be quite severe. They can bring about symptoms that are uncomfortable and cause us to be miserable. God wants us happy, active, well, and strong to perform His works and our purpose here on earth. Ultimately, these adverse reactions can get in the way of us fulfilling our God-given purpose. We should be aware and not allow these reactions to rob us of a wholesome life. This may involve avoiding culprit foods.

Typically, food allergies cause an immune system reaction that can affect numerous organs in the body and result in a range of symptoms. Some of these allergies can cause extreme discomfort or be life-threatening. Conversely, food intolerance symptoms are generally less serious and are often limited to digestive problems.[1]

Let's look at the most common food culprits.

### Gluten[2]

Gluten is a composite of proteins that is stored together with starch and is found in various cereal grains such as wheat, oats, rye, and barley. It is also found in products derived from these grains such as breads, pastas, beer, soy sauce, and as a supplemental protein addition in many vegetarian meals. Gluten can also be used as a stabilizing agent in foods such as ice cream and ketchup. Gluten supplies 75-85% of the total protein in foods that contain it.

In a small percentage of individuals, gluten can trigger adverse autoimmune reactions. Many people who think that they are allergic to gluten find out that they really are not. They are simply reacting to all the junk present in improperly grown foods and not to gluten. When these individuals eat grains grown free of GMOs for instance, they do not suffer any adverse reactions. GMOs have brought about increased incidents of allergies.[3]

Adverse reactions to gluten include celiac disease, dermatitis, psoriasis, bloating, diarrhea, abdominal pain, and headaches.[4] The allergy causes the immune system to respond abnormally to gluten and treat it as a threatening foreign body. These conditions are typically treated with a gluten-free diet.

A serious autoimmune disease triggered by gluten ingestion is gluten ataxia. It can cause damage in the balance centre of the brain—the cerebellum. Let's take a closer look at celiac disease and gluten ataxia, as they can have far-reaching effects on what we eat and how we feel.

For people with celiac disease, eating gluten triggers an immune response in their small intestine.[5] Over time, this reaction damages the small intestine's lining and prevents absorption of some nutrients (malabsorption). Symptoms include diarrhea, weight loss, and fatigue. These are the most common symptoms. Symptoms that are more serious include anemia and bloating and can lead to serious complications. Other symptoms unrelated to the digestive system include headaches, fatigue, mouth ulcers, acid reflux and heartburn, dermatitis, and joint pain.

The signs and symptoms of celiac disease vary greatly in individuals. There is no cure for celiac disease. Most people can help manage symptoms and promote healing in their intestines by following a strict gluten-free diet.

People with gluten ataxia[6] can show signs of imbalance in their speech, gait, and have problems swallowing food. Early diagnosis here is key in order to prevent its progression. The effectiveness of treatment, which is with a gluten-free diet, is dependent on how much time has passed between the onset of ataxia and its diagnosis. This is so because neuron death in the cerebellum due to gluten exposure is irreversible.

A big problem with gluten is its unexpected presence in foods like ketchup and ice cream, such as mentioned above. Hidden gluten can constitute a hazard for people sensitive to gluten.

## Lactose[7]

Many people have difficulty digesting lactose, a sugar found in milk. This inability is referred to as lactose intolerance and is usually caused by a deficiency of an enzyme in the body called lactase. This condition is characterized by one or multiple symptoms such as bloating, gas, diarrhea, and stomach pain.

Lactose intolerance can develop at any age and can be triggered by other conditions such as Chron's disease.[8] The intolerance to lactose is usually self-diagnosable, can last for years, or be lifelong. It cannot be cured but can be managed by avoiding products that contain lactose. I gravitated toward lactose free milk as I became somewhat lactose intolerant in my early 50s. There are now many lactose-free dairy products sold in grocery stores, including many unsweetened substitutes like almond, oatmeal and hazelnut "milks." Interestingly I have only had a problem with dairy milk, not its related products like yogurt, cheese and ice cream. However, I am trying to stay away from dairy products as I learn more about them. I discussed this in *Chapter 2*.

## Nuts[9]

A growing number of people are allergic to nuts. The term "nut allergy" can be confusing, as it is typically used to describe an allergic reaction to the fruit of unrelated plants such as peanuts, seeds, and other nuts that grow on trees. Peanuts are legumes; tree nuts include almonds, cashews, macadamia nuts, and walnuts. Seeds include sesame seeds and sunflower seeds.

Peanut allergy is one of the most common allergies of this range of allergies. People who are allergic to peanuts will not necessarily be allergic to almonds, cashew and macadamia nuts, or seeds. The most common symptom of these allergies is the appearance of hives, which are raised reddish bumps on the skin. These can be quite unpleasant and often cause discomfort depending on their location in the body.

I once had an allergy to peanuts develop on the back of my knee, and so wearing trousers, fitted skirts and dresses, and even sitting were all quite uncomfortable. This caused me to have to eliminate these nuts that had previously been an integral part of my diet.

Allergic symptoms to this group of foods can also be a runny nose, nausea or vomiting, and cramps. Other allergies can be life-threatening. Peanuts, tree nuts, and seeds are some of the most common food triggers for life-threatening, severe allergic reactions. For the purposes of this book, I will not dwell too much on these extreme allergies, except to remind us to pay attention to food labels, especially if we are allergic to these foods.

I bring to your attention the case of a teenager who died after eating a baguette sandwich that had sesame seeds.[10] She was allergic to these seeds. Unfortunately, there was no allergen advice on the sandwich wrapper. Most food labels and restaurants now provide specific information about nuts, seeds, and other allergens, going as far as stating if their produce was prepared in an environment free/or not from nuts, seeds, etc.

These allergies can sometimes develop suddenly. If it is a relatively mild reaction like hives, the culprit food can be determined by initially paying attention to the timing of the allergic symptoms and avoiding the food for a time and then reintroducing it. If the symptoms stop and return, then we probably are allergic to it. Other more serious symptoms will need medical attention, such as a diagnosis by an allergy specialist.

## Seafood[11]

The types of seafood that can cause allergies include scaly fish, and shellfish such as oysters, mussels, squid, prawns, and crayfish. The symptoms of allergies to seafood generally develop very quickly, within minutes of consuming foods with these ingredients, and up to two hours after. In some cases, after the first symptoms go away, a second wave of symptoms can appear one to two hours later.

There are various symptoms which may include itching or eczema and hives. Another serious reaction is anaphylaxis, which causes swelling of the face, lips, throat, and tongue. Swelling in the latter two can make breathing difficult and be life-threatening. Other symptoms include tingling in the mouth, nausea, diarrhea, abdominal pain, vomiting, nasal congestion, and wheezing. Mild allergic reactions to seafood can be treated with antihistamines. More severe allergies may require an emergency injection.

The most severe food allergy reactions are to peanuts, tree nuts, such as cashews and almonds, seeds, shellfish, and fish. Typically, food allergies last a lifetime and tend to be more severe if an individual is asthmatic.

## Managing Food Allergens

The best way to manage allergies to gluten, peanuts, other nuts, seeds, seafood, and all other allergens is to avoid all products containing these ingredients. However, even when we are careful, it can often be a Herculean task avoiding all contact with these foods. Sometimes these culprits can appear when least expected. If we are unfortunate enough to suffer from adverse reactions to foods, we must pay extra attention to food labels, particularly if these symptoms are life-threatening.

When food labels are unavailable, say at a dinner party, barbecue, etc., we should always make enquiries before eating if there are any foods that are known to cause us adverse reactions. It will also be wise to let your host know of any food allergies in advance.[12]

As mentioned above, many restaurants and other food outlets now provide warnings about foods containing nuts, seeds, and other well-known food allergy culprits. This is imperative as some of these allergies can be life-threatening.

# Chapter 10

# Cannot Seem to Lose Weight?

When you have been honest with yourself, have eaten mindfully, exercised well, but are still struggling, and finding it difficult or even impossible to lose weight, you may need to take a look at other factors that could be a problem.

## Sleep

Sleep is very important, indeed essential, to our general well-being. It is also vital when we are trying to lose weight. It is probably as crucial a factor as diet and exercise. There is mounting evidence that shows that sleep may be the missing factor for many people who are struggling to lose weight.[1] A minimum of 7 hours of quality sleep is recommended. Studies have found that inadequate sleep can lead to weight gain and a higher likelihood of obesity in both children and adults.

We need to learn to make our bedrooms conducive for quality sleep. For many, a quiet, pleasant temperature and dark environment are essential. I personally cannot sleep with the TV or music on and prefer a pitch-dark room.

Sleep deprivation affects the hormones that regulate hunger and appetite. The hormone leptin curbs appetite by regulating satiety/fullness.Sleep deprivation reduces leptin, and so leads to an increase in appetite, particularly carb and sugar cravings, the next day. Temptations may then become hard to resist and portion sizes difficult to control. This can contribute to weight gain.

Another hormone that is affected by sleep deprivation is the hunger hormone, ghrelin. Sleep deprivation causes this hormone to increase,[2] resulting in overeating and therefore weight gain. Increased eating may also simply be from an increase in the number of hours spent awake. This is especially detrimental when this time is spent inactive, such as slouched on a couch watching television.

Insufficient sleep can result in daytime fatigue and can reduce the likelihood and motivation to exercise. We are also more likely to tire easily during physical activity when we are sleep deprived. On the other hand, getting sufficient sleep should help improve our athletic performance and its benefits. Remember as discussed in Chapter 8, exercise can be a contributory factor in losing and maintaining weight loss. The effect of insufficient sleep as it relates to resistance to insulin is also discussed below.

With sleep deprivation, a vicious cycle can easily ensue. The less we sleep, the more weight we gain, and the more weight we gain, the harder it is to sleep well. Adequate sleep also helps lower stress and has anti-inflammatory properties; it facilitates the loss of a lot of body fluids...so chronic inflammation goes down. Our body heals, recovers, and rebuilds itself when we sleep.

We should not go to bed with an empty stomach as it may prevent us from falling asleep soundly. Gorging before sleep is also not a good idea. It will likely disrupt our sleep, too. I find that eating a light dinner at a time that allows at least 3-3 ½ hours before a regular bedtime helps me get a good night's sleep. Say, for example, that bedtime is at 10 p.m.; we should try to ensure that we have finished dinner by 6.30-7 p.m. A regular bedtime is really helpful to ensure adequate sleep. Of course, there can be exceptions.

### The Dreaded Weight Loss Plateau

Have you found that when on a weight loss regimen, the weight sometimes comes off rapidly in the beginning, and then there is little or no progress? This can be frustrating and discouraging and is referred to as a weight loss plateau. The following are some strategies to ensure continued progress in your weight loss efforts:[3]

### Tweak Your Carbs Intake

Try reducing your carb intake for a while. A reduced carb intake will cause our bodies to produce ketones, which have been shown to cause weight loss. This is what causes people on the keto diet to lose weight quickly. Remember, though, that we questioned the sustainability of this method of weight loss in Chapter 2. I only recommend a highly reduced carb intake for a very short while. I would say no more than 2 weeks at a time. I do however recommend a rule of little or no carbs after 4 p.m. on regular basis. I discussed this more extensively in *Chapter 4*.

### Increase Protein Intake

It is generally not a good idea to skimp on protein and particularly not when one is experiencing an undesired weight plateau. As discussed in Chapter 7, protein reduces hunger, boosts metabolism, and prevents muscle loss. These will all encourage weight loss.

### Increase Your Veggies

Veggies are always the ideal food for weight loss and at other times, as they are typically low in calories and high in fiber. They can be and are a good idea eaten at every meal.

### Fiber

Including more fiber in your diet may help you break through a weight loss plateau. This is especially true with soluble fiber, the type that dissolves in water or other liquids. This fiber slows down the movement of food through our digestive tract, which can help us feel full and satisfied for longer periods. Foods that contain soluble fiber include carrots, apples, oats, peas, beans, and citrus fruit.

### Coffee, Tea, and Water

Coffee, green tea, and water can help boost our metabolic rate and assist with weight loss. These have all been discussed in Chapter 7.

### Be Active

Increase exercise frequency and/or intensity. This may help reverse a weight loss plateau. This is because our metabolic rate can slow down as we lose weight. Exercise is important, as is our level of activity throughout the day. They both influence the number of calories we burn each day. Exercise and activity were discussed extensively in Chapter 8.

### Manage Stress

Stress often causes weight loss plateaus and can trigger food cravings and comfort eating. Comfort eating and food cravings are likely to cause more than plateaus...weight gain. Stress also increases our body's production of cortisol, which is known as the "stress hormone." It helps our body respond to stress, but it can also increase fat storage around our midsection. This effect seems to be stronger in women. High levels of cortisol can make weight loss very difficult.

### Get Plenty Sleep

Good quality sleep is non-negotiable for good mental, emotional, and physical health. Not getting adequate sleep may be a contributing factor in cases of weight loss plateaus. The importance of sleep was discussed more extensively earlier in this chapter.

## Scales

Oftentimes, scale readings may not accurately reflect our progress. It is not easy to be well-informed about changes in our body composition using only scales. If we are working out regularly, we could be building muscle and losing fat yet maintaining a stable weight. Our goal should be centered more on fat loss rather than on weight loss. This popular weight loss gauge is discussed further in *Chapter 12*.

## Be Accountable About What You Eat

Above all we must be mindful about what we eat. We should not underestimate the amount of food we eat. Oftentimes we consume more food than we think. I discuss closet eating in the next chapter.

What can we do if we do not see progress after eating and exercising mindfully, sleeping well, and dealing with what was thought to be a weight loss plateau? There could be an undiagnosed and therefore untreated condition(s), and we may need to see a doctor.

There are some conditions that can hinder our ability to lose weight, despite mindfully eating, exercising, and sleeping well. Some of these could be resistance to insulin, Cushing's Syndrome, and the thyroid condition, hypothyroidism. These conditions, among others, can make weight loss almost impossible without diagnosis and treatment.

## Resistance to Insulin[4]

Insulin resistance causes our body to respond abnormally to the insulin hormone. Insulin is produced in the pancreas and helps control the amount of sugar (glucose) in the blood. Over time, this causes our blood sugar levels to rise. This aberration can set one up for type 2 diabetes, as well as heart disease.

A lack of exercise, smoking, and even skimping on sleep can increase excess body weight and belly fat and are significant contributors to this condition. Genetics, aging, and ethnicity can also play roles in developing insulin resistance.

Let's take a closer look at sleep, as it relates to this condition. Deprivation of sleep can increase the production of cortisol. This can make cells more resistant to insulin. Lack of sleep can also trigger changes to other hormones such as the testosterone- and thyroid-stimulating hormone (TSH), which can lead to decreased insulin sensitivity and therefore higher blood glucose.

Signs of insulin resistance include:[5]

- extreme thirst or hunger
- feeling hungry even after a meal
- increased or frequent urination
- tingling sensations in hands or feet
- feeling more tired than usual
- frequent infections
- evidence in blood work

Insulin resistance can make it hard to lose weight. This hormone does far more than control our blood sugar levels: it also controls fat storage. This condition is the main reason why so many people struggle to lose weight, and not because they are idle or greedy.

## Treatment

Insulin resistance can be reversed through aggressive lifestyle changes. The foods that will cure this malady are nutrient-dense vegetables, fruits, whole grains, fish, and lean poultry and other lean meats. It is necessary to avoid refined sugars, unhealthy fats, fatty meats, processed starches, and other processed foods and drinks. An exercise regime will also be beneficial.

## Gut Health

I include here a very brief discussion on gut health. The condition of our gut has an enormous impact on our overall health. It can be the reason why weight just does not seem to shift. Gut health refers to the function and balance of bacteria in our gastrointestinal tract. When our gut is healthy, our stomach, intestines and other organs all work together to enable us to eat and digest food without discomfort. When our gut health is compromised, it can cause inflammation, which can lead to increased fat storage. It can also cause poor nutrient absorption from the foods we consume.[6]

A leaky gut[7] is an unhealthy gut condition in which bacteria and toxins are able to flow through the intestinal wall into our bloodstream. This can lead to many adverse conditions including:

- fatigue
- headaches
- confusion
- joint pain
- skin problems such as acne and eczema flare ups
- chronic diarrhea and constipation

**How to Improve Gut Health**[8]

Eating foods that contribute to a healthy gut microbiome is essential. This includes:

- Reducing the consumption of processed, high-sugar, and fatty foods.

- Eating plenty of plant-based foods such as fresh vegetables and fruits.

- For people who eat meat, lean protein such as chicken and fish are healthier than red meats. Nuts, seeds and legumes like beans and lentils are also excellent sources of both protein and fiber.

- A diet high in fiber is also essential for a healthy gut.

- Quality sleep may be essential for gut health. Oftentimes people with disturbed sleep patterns have digestive concerns.

- Regular exercise reduces stress levels and helps maintain a healthy weight. These will have a positive effect on gut health.

- Stop the unnecessary use of antibiotics, as they can wipe out both bad and good bacteria in the gut. Many consume antibiotics for conditions such as the common cold or a sore throat. These are usually viral infections and do not respond to antibiotics anyway.

As we can now see, an unhealthy gut can also affect our wellness and ability to lose weight.

**Cushing's Syndrome**[9]

Cushing's Syndrome is caused by a prolonged exposure to cortisol, a stress hormone. It is a big public health enemy. Elevated cortisol levels can interfere with learning and memory, lower immune function, and bone density. It can increase weight, cholesterol, and blood pressure, and cause heart disease, to name a few.

This ailment can be the result of an excessive ingestion of cortisol-like medication such as prednisone, or a tumor, which causes or results in the adrenal gland producing excessive cortisol. Signs and symptoms may include rapid weight gain, especially around the midsection. I know a lady who put on nearly 22.4 pounds (10 kg.) in six months. Other symptoms are high blood pressure, fatty deposits around the face and upper back, excess sweating, and fat loss from arms and legs. Occasionally, it can result in changes to the sufferer's mood, chronic lethargy, and headaches. It can also cause women to have irregular periods and increased coarse body hair growth.

The diagnosis of this syndrome is made by a doctor and typically involves some steps. Generally, the first step is to check the individual's medication. In the second step, cortisol levels are measured in the urine, saliva, or in the blood. If the diagnosis finds prescribed medications to be a culprit, they can be slowly stopped. If caused by a tumor, treatment may be a combination of surgery, chemotherapy, and/or radiotherapy. It is more common in people who are 20-50 years of age and occurs three times more often in women than in men. The prognosis of this condition is generally good with treatment.

For people with Cushing's Syndrome, chronic stress can increase the risk for depression and mental illness and can lead ultimately to a lower life expectancy. People with this condition must learn to de-stress. Indeed, we all do. This reduces cortisol levels. Below are a few de-stressing techniques.

## Regular Physical Activity

Activities like kickboxing or the use of a punching bag are great ways to de-stress. These activities let out aggression (without hurting anyone), thus reducing cortisol.

Aerobic activities such as walking, jogging, biking, swimming, or riding the elliptical trainer are other great ways to burn up cortisol. As little as 20 to 30 minutes of these activities 4-5 days per week goes a long way to lowering this hormone.

Fear increases cortisol. Regular physical activity decreases fear by increasing our self-confidence and resilience and reducing cortisol.[10]

## Saunas[11]

A sauna is a room with dry heat. They have been used for thousands of years and are still popular today. They are useful in helping people unwind and relax. The heat in a sauna causes our heart rate to increase and blood vessels to widen. This increase and improves circulation in much the same way as low to moderate exercise can do depending on the time spent in the sauna. The improved circulation may also promote relaxation. This can lead to improved feelings of well-being and reduced cortisol levels.

## Hypothyroidism[12]

Hypothyroidism is a thyroid condition, that is more common in women. The thyroid is a small gland in the front of our neck. It is our "energy gland." When it is operating properly, we have lots of energy and can be active. Conversely, when it is not, it can leave us feeling out of sorts.

Unexplained weight gain may be the result of low levels of thyroid hormones. This is hypothyroidism. Conversely, if the thyroid produces more hormones than the body requires, it can result in unexpected weight loss known as hyperthyroidism. Hypothyroidism is far more common, and I will focus only on this condition for the purpose of this book.

Low thyroid hormone levels can cause sudden weight gain, especially around the waistline. When an individual develops hypothyroidism, there is a slowdown in metabolism. This causes the rate at which the body burns food to slow down, resulting in weight gain ranging from between 10 and 30 pounds (4.54 - 13.62 kg). Most of this extra weight is due to water and salt.[13] This condition can be quite frustrating, as weight can be gained even with reduced food consumption. Hypothyroidism can cause a decrease in appetite while there is still an increase in weight. Loss of this weight is often an uphill struggle if left untreated.[14] With hypothyroidism, one can feel like energy, happiness, and youth are being sucked away.

Other common signs of an under active thyroid include:[15]

- Extreme fatigue, which can be as bad as waking up tired and going to sleep tired. Some may find it difficult getting out of bed in the morning and barely being able to function by afternoon;

- Unexplained weight gain;

- Brain fog. This can make concentrating on various tasks more difficult and certainly more so than in the past;

- Irritability and depression. This includes mood swings and a struggle with bouts of anxiety;

- Digestive problems. These can include constipation, bloating, and chronic gas;

- Increased cholesterol levels;

- A slower heart rate;

- Loss of memory;

- Dry or brittle hair.

It can be easy to overlook thyroid symptoms and feel stuck with lifelong fatigue, weight gain and just generally feeling under the weather. This is especially so if doctors and family tell you "you're fine" and "it's all in your head."

The way I see it, if you are honestly eating well, exercising, not feeling well, and are tired and putting on weight, do not let anyone convince you that you are imagining things. Insist on medical checks to find out what the problem could be.

### Treatment[16]

The treatment for hypothyroidism is three-pronged, involving not only medication but a diet overhaul and exercise regimen to lose weight and improve general well-being.

The weight associated with hypothyroidism can often be stabilized by taking daily hormone tablets to replace the hormones not being produced by the thyroid. In order to avoid being saddled with the excess pounds gained before diagnosis and treatment, sufferers often require a weight-loss diet as well as an exercise routine. The increased activity can raise metabolism, burn fat, reduce blood sugar levels, and balance leptin. The hormone leptin curbs appetite and so promotes weight loss.

Another condition that can make weight loss difficult is obesity, especially when related to hormones.

### Obesity

Obesity can make weight loss difficult, particularly when related to hormone levels.[17] I am not discussing hormone induced obesity. Obesity is a disorder that involves excessive body fat and increases the risk of health problems.

This excess fat can be under the skin (subcutaneous) and visceral fat around organs. The latter can be very dangerous and is discussed further later on.

Obesity often results from the prolonged consumption of excessive amounts of unhealthy foods, more than are burned by normal daily activities including exercise. This type of obesity resulting from excessive food and lack of exercise can be prevented by societal changes and personal choices. Preventive measures will include making a change in diet and exercise, minimizing the consumption of ultra-processed foods and becoming more active. These are effective strategies for obesity prevention and treatment. In extreme cases surgery may be recommended.

Abdominal fat or visceral fat[18] refers to excess weight that develops over time around the abdominal cavity. It is also known as "active fat" since it influences how hormones function in the body. It can have potentially dangerous consequences. As visceral fat is in the abdominal cavity, it is close to many vital organs such as the pancreas, liver, and intestines. The higher the amount of visceral fat a person stores, the more at risk they are for certain health complications such as type 2 diabetes and heart disease.

Typical causes of this condition include an unhealthy diet, a sedentary lifestyle, and/or alcohol use. It can be controlled and even reduced by eating a healthy diet rich in vegetables, fruits, and whole grains. It may also help to avoid saturated fats and big meal portions.

Adapting a moderate aerobic activity of at least 150 minutes per week helps to increase weight loss and is also very beneficial. Medical care should be sought in extreme cases. As a rule, a man with a waist measurement exceeding 40 inches (about 102 cm) and a woman with a waist measurement above 35 inches (89 cm) should be concerned.

Obesity can very adversely affect one's confidence and, in extreme cases, hinder one from achieving God's purpose. It can be such a crippling, demoralizing experience for some that it causes sufferers to become very reclusive. Thankfully, there is often a solution. Sometimes people just need to take responsibility and get a hold of their bad eating habits. You will see in **Chapter 11**that we can have help to do this.

Some individuals are predisposed to severe obesity. However, lifestyle interventions can be effective in many of these people. It is often not enough to say an individual is genetically wired to be obese. Genes do not have to result in obesity if an intentional decision with food and exercise, is taken.[19] There is usually a specific reason for weight increase and often proven remedies to tackle this malaise. Only some of these have been discussed in this chapter.

# Chapter 11

# Losing Weight

Our quest for healthy living may prove arduous when we start, as old habits such as a long-sustained, sedentary lifestyle and reckless eating can be hard to break. It is unlikely to be a quick fix. In addition, if we have been addicted to junk food and drinks, we will need time to wean ourselves off them. We will likely have withdrawal symptoms similar to that suffered by a drug addict. This is still no reason to say we cannot do it. If we get our minds right, our bodies will eventually toe the line.[1]

We need perseverance over time to be successful with losing weight. Remember that we do not have to struggle by ourselves to be successful here. God is very detailed about ALL that concerns us. We can therefore ask the Holy Spirit for help if we are desirous and committed to losing and keeping weight off and are struggling. We must never, ever say we cannot lose weight and keep it off, especially if we are otherwise healthy. We can. God promises us in:

**Philippians 4:13 AMPC**
*I have strength for all things in Christ Who empowers me [I am ready for anything and equal to anything through Him Who infuses inner strength into me; I am self-sufficient in Christ's sufficiency].*

I recently had the opportunity to advise a lady trying to lose weight and keep it off. I told her to remember that she could do all things through Christ who strengthens her. She believed and it worked for her. She is now in the maintenance phase and has been for months...enjoying her slimmer, healthier body. It will work for you, too, if you believe, are intentional with what you eat, and exercise.

Remember also:

**Psalms 37:4-5 KJV**
*Delight thyself also in the Lord; and he shall give thee the desires of thine heart. Commit thy way unto the Lord; trust also in him; and he shall bring it to pass.*

It is always productive including Him in all that we do. Let's look at more scripture.

**Matthew 7:7-8 KJV**
*Ask, and it shall be given you; seek, and ye shall find; knock, and it shall be opened unto you: For every one that asketh receiveth; and he that seeketh findeth; and to him that knocketh it shall be opened.*

**Ephesians 3:20 TPT**
*Never doubt God's mighty power to work in you and accomplish all this. He will achieve infinitely more than your greatest request, your most unbelievable dream, and exceed your wildest imagination! He will outdo them all, for his miraculous power constantly energizes you.*

As I have said, it may be difficult but certainly not impossible to make the changes we want to make. Our intention to adopt a healthy lifestyle is good, but we may fail several times. Remember that we battle against the flesh. We must learn to trust God. The Holy Spirit is God's power within us to defeat our flesh. We can ask the Holy Spirit for help with conquering our flesh.[2]

It is not too difficult to live a healthy life. It is what God wants us to do; it involves looking after our body—His temple. He equips us with the Grace to do this. His yoke is easy.

**Matthew 11:30 KJV**
*For my yoke is easy, and my burden is light.*

We must choose to trust and let Him help us step away from old, unhealthy tendencies and develop new habits that will enable us to take hold of a healthier, more fulfilling life.[3]

Our health and wellness are intertwined. We are at our optimum when our physical body, heart, mind, and emotions are all healthy. Living well will require us being attentive to all these facets of our life.[4] Let us honor God with the healthy choices we make, so that we can experience all that God has for us, by fulfilling ALL that God has planned for our lives including our purpose. His mighty power works within us to accomplish all He wants us to. Our part is to surrender, to trust, and to obey.[5]

When I initially lost weight, I did not have the relationship I now have with the Lord. There were times then when I had major setbacks; I would have binges. Fortunately, I never put back on all the weight I lost. Those times were always linked to periods when I was going through trials. For some people weight loss accompanies their trials as they lose their appetite. Mine was always the opposite, an unhealthy relationship with food and binge-ing, which was quickly followed by weight gain.

My experience with food since my closer walk with the Lord has been different and very stable. In 2017, when my dear husband, John A. Jones, passed away, I did not have any binges. I leaned totally on God. It was only because of my TOTAL trust in God and dependence on Him that I did not ever turn to food as a crutch during this very trying period. I have no doubt in my mind that I would have used food as a crutch if I had had this experience 25 or so years ago.

Now let us not forget that there is nothing wrong in indulging every now and again. We must make it an exception rather than the rule though. In life we are faced with choices every day, right and wrong. It is certainly the case with the foods we choose to eat on a regular basis. We have a choice to eat foods that nourish our bodies or not.

We must also not be closet eaters. These individuals typically do not eat in public. They typically eat surreptitiously while they cook and when alone, with very little food eaten when with others. This often causes people to wonder how they can eat so little and yet struggle with their weight. We must realize that whatever and whenever we eat, our bodies absorb the food. This happens whether we do it in the open or behind closed doors. I say it directly like this because of the many surreptitious eaters out there. Whether you eat in public or privately—you have eaten. Closet eating is an eating disorder. Registered Psychotherapists can provide help with overcoming it.[6]

We should also not take pleasure in eating thoughtlessly. We must try to be intentional and accountable about what, when, and how much we eat. When out at parties, restaurants, etc., and are faced with a wide array of foods, we must be disciplined. We do not have to eat all that we are offered, or all that is available.

Your healthy lifestyle will not look exactly like mine. It will be unique to you. There are universal rules about health that we all need to work within; but the day-to-day specifics of what we eat, how we exercise, how we make time to rest, will be unique to each of us. We must keep these specifics conducive to our long-term goals, focus on small steps every day, and watch our lives transform.[7]

God gave us life so that we can make a difference. When we choose to neglect our health and end up sick, struggling to get through each day, we rarely have much impact on the world. Dead people have even less, and often none at all. By deciding to get healthy, we are taking a major step towards maximizing the difference our lives can make now and for generations to come. We are choosing to step away from the patterns and habits that have harmed our health. And choose to head towards the life we were made for:[8] a healthy one with which we can fulfill God's perfect will.

We are here for a purpose and have an impact to make on others. We should not let a lack of discipline in our eating and exercise patterns, and therefore the quality of our health, sabotage the fullness of the life we were intended for. Our family, friends, community, and the church are all good reasons to take care of ourselves,[9] as our health also directly affects those dear and close to us.

Let us learn to give of ourselves from a place of strength and wholeness. We must steward our body so that we can love our God, others, and ourselves fully.[10]

I cannot emphasize enough that we must be careful about letting others convince us that God is not concerned with what we eat. He is. Each one of us is His careful and unique creation. We are His hands and feet here on earth.[11] Our body is the vessel in which He resides as the Holy Spirit.

**Ephesians 2:10 KJV**
*For we are his workmanship, created in Christ Jesus unto good works, which God hath before ordained that we should walk in them.*

God has given each of us a unique gift. Your gift is different from mine. We all have distinctive skills, interests, passions, and life experiences with which to live out our purpose. He wants to put us to good use and shine through us mightily.[12] It is all up to us though, as He always gives us free will. The everyday choices we make to keep ourselves healthy are so important, both to the quality of our lives and in our ability to do all that God has planned for us.[13]

We should treat our physical bodies, His temple, with respect. We must learn to take responsibility for what, when, and the way we eat and exercise. Learn to say, "no, thank you!" when offered excessive amounts of food and/or when we are just not hungry. As I have mentioned earlier, when faced with unhealthy food choices I really like the saying, "a minute on the lips, a lifetime on the hips." That helps me keep from being consistently off-track.

We are new in Christ. Let's lay down our old lives so the new can begin.

### 2 Corinthians 5:17 KJV
*Therefore, if any man be in Christ, he is a new creature: old things are passed away; behold, all things are become new.*

Nothing you do by the power of God is too hard. We often make situations very difficult and even frustrating by trying to do things through our own strength. However, when we learn to rest in God through faith in His Word, we minimize our struggles. This is certainly applicable to our efforts of weight loss and management. I believe without any doubt that if I had known many years ago, when I embarked on my weight loss and maintenance program, to rely on God for guidance rather than solely on my own wits, it would have been a much easier journey.

No more excuses if we want to lose weight. We can. We can do all things through Christ who strengthens us. If we do not feel our best and want to be fit, develop and maintain a spring in our step, have a good attitude, and above all fulfill God's purpose for our life…we can. Not in our strength but through Him.

# Chapter 12

# Useful Tips

In this chapter I am going to share some tips I have used to keep weight off and maintain a healthy lifestyle. I have already discussed some of these points, but they are important enough to mention again. Indeed, they cannot be overemphasized.

## Processed Sugar, Foods, and Drinks

I dedicated all of Chapter 5 to processed foods and drinks. It cannot be said enough that these products must be consumed with great caution. They are responsible for so many ailments and can be detrimental to our general well-being both in the short and long term. Thankfully, there is a remedy: they should be eaten, if at all, very sparingly.

## Avoid Stress

Stress can be negative or positive. I will dwell only on negative stress. Stress is our body's reaction to any change that requires a response. The body reacts to these changes with mental, physical, and emotional responses. Stress can be internal from our body or thoughts or external from our environment. It can be caused by a physical or emotional stimulus or situation.[1] "Stress doesn't only make us feel awful emotionally. It can also exacerbate just about any health condition you can think of," according to Jay Winner, MD.

Stress should be managed, as its effects can be far-reaching, especially if its levels are high, on-going, and chronic. Chronic stress can cause or exacerbate many serious health conditions including mental health problems like anxiety and depression. Cardiovascular diseases such as high blood pressure, heart disease, heart attacks, and stroke can also be caused or made worse by stress. Some other ailments that are often related to stress are headaches, gastrointestinal problems, accelerated aging, and premature death.[2] These will invariably have a negative impact on our well-being and health.

We must never underestimate the effects of stress. Various conditions such as shingles that can affect our well-being are indirectly linked to stress. Stress does not technically cause shingles, but it can cause our immune system to weaken. A weakened immune system can put us at risk for shingles, which is a viral illness. The varicella zoster virus, the same virus responsible for chickenpox, causes shingles. It only occurs in individuals who have previously had chicken pox. Shingles typically causes a blister-like rash, which can be quite painful and itchy. It often occurs around either the left or the right side of the torso.[3]

I was in shock and stressed when my husband passed, and I came down with shingles. I was fortunate not to suffer much pain, but the blisters were quite itchy, angry looking, and caused me not to be able to sleep on my back, my preferred sleeping position. This made me quite tired as I could not get sufficient sleep for a while.

Stress has also been found to contribute to the onset of various cancers and can worsen the condition. We ought to manage our stress levels and so avoid the far-reaching consequences it can cause. We need to stop, breathe, smell the flowers, and learn to rest, or we open ourselves up to a greater risk of stress-induced ailments.

### Water

We should drink at least eight medium to large glasses of water each day; more in a hot climate and when exercising. It is also a good habit to drink it immediately we wake up and before eating our meals. Water curbs cravings, helps us stay full, and ensures a healthy, ingested food movement along our digestive systems.

We can also increase our water intake by snacking on vegetables such as carrots, cucumbers, and celery, and fruits such as berries and apples. These contain water naturally. They are also far more nutritious than popular snacks such as pretzels, crisps (potato chips), corn chips, and salted nuts (which are all quite salty).

Some people wrongly think that drinking water may be bad if one has the propensity to retain water. This is far from the truth. On the contrary, drinking more water decreases water retention. Water retention often occurs because our bodies are dehydrated. Our body goes into the conservation mode of water retention to prevent dehydration. Water is the elixir of life.

**Vitamin D**

Vitamin D,[4] like other vitamins, is important, and is one of the many nutrients needed by our body to remain healthy. It is manufactured in our skin after the absorption of sunlight. Health practitioners recommend that supplements of this vitamin be taken particularly by people of color during winter months, when there is little or no sunlight for extended periods.

Vitamin D aids the absorption of calcium in our body. Together with calcium, Vitamin D helps build bones and keeps them healthy and strong. Vitamin D is both anti-inflammatory and essential for a healthy immune system and healthy teeth, too. Deficiency in Vitamin D can cause symptoms such as thinning or brittle bones, osteoporosis, frequent bone fractures, anxiety or depression and may be responsible for some aggressive cancers in people of color.[5] All these will negatively affect our general well-being.

The Covid 19 pandemic has increased discussions on the importance of Vitamin D as it relates to the health of our immune system. Very briefly, a deficiency in Vitamin D compromises our immune system and increases an individual's susceptibility to various infections.

### Snacks[6]

Can we eat snacks? Absolutely! These are small portions of food typically eaten to stave off hunger and are not a complete meal. Snacks are generally eaten outside of the traditional meals of breakfast, lunch, and dinner and are often consumed between meals.

Snacking in the absence of hunger often leads to the consumption of readily available processed snack foods which typically have large amounts of sugar, salt, and fat. Unnecessary snacking is likely to promote weight gain and poor nutrition. Examples of snacks include fruits, nuts, leftovers, packaged snack foods, and cheese.

Over the years, I have found that I only tend to require a snack between breakfast and lunch, rarely between lunch and dinner, and almost never after dinner before bedtime. I truly believe that when we eat a wholesome meal consisting of a good variety of nutrient-dense foods, there really is no need to snack. My experience with snacking is that it is more likely to happen after exercising or when I have not eaten well. This typically happens when I have not taken the time to plan my meal or I'm on the run. Fortunately, this is not a regular occurrence with me. People who know me well are very aware how seriously I take my meals, what I eat, and when. Some find my stance quite irritating, but hey, it works...

A snack comes in handy particularly after a vigorous workout, which for me is usually between breakfast and lunch. I usually snack on nuts, yogurt, and/or fruit. I always gravitate towards berries when they are available, as they are very nutritious and have a low glycemic index. Small apples are also a good snack. The dried roasted groundnuts, popular in Nigeria, or others such as pistachios, cashew nuts, Brazil nuts, and almonds are also nutritious snacks in moderate amounts. My choice of nuts, as with all I eat, is often dependent on my location. I recently acquired a taste for dark chocolate with a high cocoa content. They tend not to be too sweet. I find a small piece for dessert after lunch is very satisfying.

We should learn to be mindful with snacking as with our regular meals. Our bodies absorb whatever we eat. We should be careful of snacking often on overly processed foods. By these, I refer to store bought biscuits, milk and white chocolate bars, cakes, muffins, ice cream, sweets, crisps, etc. There is no harm in occasionally indulging, but we must try not to overdo it. Processed foods have been discussed in detail in Chapter 5.

### Processed Sugar Versus Pure Honey[7]

Processed sugar and pure honey are two of the most used sweeteners. I will use the terms processed sugar and sugar, pure honey and honey interchangeably. They are both carbohydrates and consist primarily of glucose and fructose. The proportions of glucose and fructose in these two sweeteners are different: Sugar has 50% glucose and 50% fructose; honey has 30% glucose and 40% fructose. Pure honey also contains pollen, water, and minerals, including potassium and magnesium. It is from these additional components that honey may derive its health benefits.

Honey typically has more calories than sugar; 64 calories per tablespoon as opposed to 49 calories for sugar. However, honey is sweeter than sugar, so less is required to achieve the same level of sweetness.

Sugar is higher on the glycemic index (GI) than honey, and so can cause spikes in blood sugar levels more quickly. This is due to its higher fructose content and the absence of trace minerals. Honey is less processed than sugar, with usually only pasteurization before consumption. Raw honey is edible and may be healthier than pasteurized varieties. The dark brown variety may contain more antioxidants than light honey.

Pure honey is healthier than sugar. I have often heard people say, "I don't use sugar, I prefer honey." Copious amounts of honey are not good though. Moderation is key here too, as both can cause weight gain if used excessively.

## Alcohol

There is nothing wrong with an occasional glass of wine, beer, a cocktail, champagne, etc. Good wines are a wonderful accompaniment to a delicious meal. Thankfully, I have never been able to drink more than a glass at a time, and so have never understood those who can drink a whole bottle—and some even more—with or without a meal. Again, with alcohol, moderation is key.

I know some of you are thinking Christians should not drink alcohol. Let's look at scripture.

### Ephesians 5:18 KJV
*And be not drunk with wine, wherein is excess; but be filled with the Spirit.*

This New Testament scripture indicates that we should not be drunk with wine. This implies we can drink in moderation, not excessively.

### John 2:9-11 KJV
*When the ruler of the feast had tasted the water that was made wine, and knew not whence it was: (but the servants which drew the water knew;) the governor of the feast called the bridegroom, And saith unto him, Every man at the beginning doth set forth good wine; and when men have well drunk, then that which is worse: but thou hast kept the good wine until now. This beginning of mira-*

*cles did Jesus in Cana of Galilee, and manifested
forth his glory; and his disciples believed on him.*

It is very interesting to think that Jesus' first ever miracle
on earth involved the conversion of water to wine. He certainly would not have started His time on earth doing
something that was wrong. All that Jesus did was good. He
never did anything that was wrong in the eyes of His
Father. He only did and said what His Father told Him. I
believe He would have heard from His Father that the
conversion of water to wine for the wedding feast was
alright.

Let us look at some more scripture:

**1 Timothy 3:2-3 KJV**
*A BISHOP then must be blameless, the husband of
one wife, vigilant, sober, of good behavior, given to
hospitality, apt to teach; NOT GIVEN TO WINE,
no striker, not greedy of filthy lucre; but patient,
not a brawler, not covetous.*

**1 Timothy 3:8 KJV**
*Likewise must the DEACONS be grave, not double
tongued, not given to MUCH wine, not greedy of
filthy lucre.*

Clearly scripture does not say that all Christians should
not drink. Only the Bishop (head of a church) should not
drink. The deacon (one who assists the head of the
church) and all others can drink in moderation.

The Bible is very clear about not drinking excessive
amounts of alcohol.

**Proverbs 20:1 GNT**
*Drinking too much makes you loud and foolish.
It's stupid to get drunk.*

**Proverbs 23:29-30 KJV**
*Who hath woe? who hath sorrow? who hath conten-*
*tions? who hath babbling? who hath wounds with-*
*out cause? who hath redness of eyes? They that tar-*
*ry LONG at the wine; they that go to seek MIXED*
*wine.*

The Bible also warns against mixing alcohol. (I have highlighted words in capital letters for emphasis).

In conclusion, if we do not feel we can stop at moderate amounts of alcohol, then it may be wise to avoid italtogether. It certainly does not say in scripture that we must all not drink alcohol. As discussed in Chapter 1, our bodies are not our own but are the temple of the Holy Ghost. We must be respectful and not abuse our bodies with excessive amounts of alcohol or anything else. Simply put, drunkenness is a sin, not moderate drinking.

**Cheat Days[8]**

These are days that are planned and typically involve a temporary break from stipulated diet rules or regular eating plans with foods/drinks that have been avoided and are usually unhealthy choices. The food/drinks consumed on these days are often quite rich, sweet, high in fat and salt, and usually in excessive amounts. In my opinion we should not plan such days, as they typically do more harm than good. It really is not a good idea to decide ahead of time that at the weekend we are going to eat pancakes, brownies, ice cream, and movie theatre popcorn, etc. What is likely to happen is that when that time comes, even if we do not feel so inclined, we are likely to eat them anyway, just because we told ourselves we could.

When faced with something that is too good to pass up, too special and sentimental, too important culturally, or simply too delicious, we should make conscious, deliberate choices as to whether or not we are going to indulge.

Remember that there is nothing wrong with indulging every now and then. We must do so mindfully though.

When we choose to indulge, we should take our time and savor every bite and eat only as much as we need to satisfy our taste buds. It may be a couple of biscuits or more. However, if we find we need a whole packet of usually up to 15-20 biscuits at a time to be satisfied, perhaps we need to check ourselves; more self-control is required. I cannot say it enough...moderation is key.

We may find that we indulge once every few weeks or while on vacation. That is okay, we just need to make conscious, deliberate decisions and be aware of our choices.[9] We must try not to overindulge and not beat ourselves up too much when we do. When we have indulged, we should quickly return to a normal healthy eating plan.

I find that remembering the saying "a minute on the lips, a lifetime on the hips" stops me from overindulging often. I guess that for men the saying could be "a minute on the lips, a lifetime around the abdomen area." These are very general statements and so should not be treated as a "be all and end all," only as a good reminder.

## Where to Eat

When we sit down to eat, it is preferable to do so at a dining table and not on a couch watching TV. It is also not a good idea to form the habit of eating on the run in a car. Rushing our food intake is also not good, as it can affect our digestive system. I sometimes feel a tightness in my stomach if I have eaten too quickly. In addition, we should try not to be distracted by our computers or the television. This can cause us to lose focus and not be mindful of the amount of food consumed. We should learn to savor our food and not gulp it down. Enjoy the process.

## Calories

This book would be incomplete without some discussion about calories. Calories are a measure of the energy in food depicted by the number of kcals (kilocalories) present in a portion of food/drink and popularized by Wilbur Atwater in the 1800s. Its use is deeply entrenched into food systems all over the world, and it is now impossible to find food labels without figures indicating the number of calories present in a container or specified portion.

For more than a century, many have used the calculation of these numbers as the universal measurement in weight loss and subsequent management. However, many calorie-focused diets fail and so are generally misleading. These failures can happen even when combined with a strict exercise regime. According to Peter Wilson in The Economist's Intelligence Podcast, May 10, 2019, calorie figures on labels are usually wrong. So also, are the numbers recorded by exercise machines. They are often unreliable.[10]

I do not generally count calories. I have learned to be more concerned about the quality of what I eat. I favor nutrient-dense foods that are real, (not overly processed) healthy, wholesome, and filling. I am super cautious with processed sugars. See Chapters 4 and 5.

Thankfully, it is not only about calories but also about how the foods that we eat interact in our bodies. More important than keeping tabs on these figures is being aware that processed sugar is very different from protein, from fat, and other carbohydrates. We will do ourselves a lot of good keeping a watchful eye on processed sugars which can be ubiquitous. Many low-fat foods count on the introduction of sugar,[11] salt, and starch to help improve the taste lost by reducing fat. These foods are therefore unlikely toeffectively aid in weight loss because of these added ingredients, as one would expect, despite being low in fat.

It is now universally known that fat is less of a demon for weight loss and maintenance than is processed sugar. This was discussed in Chapter 5. The most effective food plan for weight loss and maintenance is one that includes natural, nutrient-dense foods, like vegetables, healthy lean meats, fruits, whole grains, nuts and seeds, and minimizes processed foods. This combination of healthy foods is more crucial for weight loss and its maintenance than a calorie count; indeed, they really are not that important when we are eating healthy. Healthy foods are filling and satisfying and make it easy to keep a healthful watch on foods consumed.

## Food Labels

We should pay attention to the nutrition labels on food packaging. These labels give information on the food's ingredients. It is particularly wise to keep a close watch on processed sugar, salt (sodium), and hydrogenated or partially hydrogenated oil.[12]

We must be mindful that sugar in foods can be in many forms. Some of these are corn syrup, sucrose, fructose, fruit juice concentrates, molasses, dried cane syrup, dehydrated cane juice, dextrose, and maltose (malt sugar).[13] They all contain processed sugars. These are low-quality carbs and can wreak havoc on our blood sugar levels. Typically, if these appear high on the list of ingredients, the food contains a high percentage of low-quality carbs that can cause our blood sugar levels to spike. The same rule applies for fats, salt, and other ingredients. The ingredients first listed will often occur in the highest concentrations in the product.

The nutritional analysis is far more beneficial than the number of calories in a product. We must skim labels for the keywords that equate to "poison." HFCS (High Fructose Corn Syrup) and Hydrogenated Oil will be high on the list of "poisonous" ingredients. Avoid foods with these ingredients or eat them sparingly. Common culprits are chips, candy, cookies, "butter-like" spreads, and microwavable popcorn.

I cannot emphasize it enough: a diet with a high percentage of nutrient-dense real foods and not processed foods is required to maintain a healthy lifestyle. Nurgul Fitzgerald, an Associate Professor in the Department of Nutritional Sciences at Rutgers University, recommends reviewing the back of a package of ready-made food. "Look at the ingredients list. Do you understand all those ingredients that go into your foods?" He suggests that we buy only those products "with the least number of ingredients and with ingredients you understand."

Other food labels we should pay attention to are those marked "organic" and "fortified."[14] Organic foods are the product of a farming practice that avoids the use of man-made pesticides, fertilizers, genetically modified organisms, (GMOs), etc. These foods are healthier than non-organic produce. Beware though of so-called organic produce, and indeed other crops whichare harvested before they are ripe and sprayed and are treated with various chemicals to keep them fresh and help them ripen. For the most part, these are packaged and transported for consumption miles away from their source. By the time these crops reach their destination, they are certainly not fresh. It is always best to buy and eat local produce in season. When we do this, we guarantee that the produce we consume is fresh and at its best both taste and nutrition-wise.[15] For example, if you live in Nigeria you will not be eating fresh organic kiwi fruit or berries like blueberries, blackberries, and raspberries, as they are not locally grown.

Organic foods are generally more expensive because they require greater labor input. Another reason for the higher costs of these foods is the limited quantities produced, which keeps the unit cost high.[16] In the case of organic animal produce, it is the grass-fed, freely roaming, and as wild as possible variety that is best.[17]

Healthily farmed crops and animals are real food that are minimally processed and do not need to be fortified. These foods are in their best state. Beware of foods and drinks labelled "fortified." These are often food products that have been stripped of some of their nutrients. There is then an attempt to "replace" some of these nutrients. As an example, freshly squeezed organic oranges are nutritious and do not require fortification. Conversely, many processed varieties are fortified with various vitamins and minerals. Imagine buying orange juice "fortified" with Vitamin C. Freshly squeezed, well-grown, and tree-ripened oranges produce a juice that is naturally rich in Vitamin C. Fortification can be a gimmick to increase the price. Eat real food the way God intended. It does not need to be fortified.[18]

God loves us so much and provides whatever is in season and grown locally to meet our nutritional needs.[19]

**Bathroom Scales**

These are a useful tool but are not the best indicator of success when losing or maintaining weight. Scales may not be our friend all the time if we think a reduction in the numbers when we weigh ourselves is the ultimate measure of progress. If we are working out regularly, we may be building muscle, which is denser than fat and weighs more. This will likely cause an increase in weight or no significant movement on our scales. Remember that we discussed in Chapter 7 that increased muscle mass equals higher metabolism, which is good. Rather than weight loss, our goal should be fat loss.[20] This will cause us to be leaner, and our clothes are likely to fit better.

In my opinion a visual approach is a more meaningful gauge of how effective our efforts are when trying to lose or maintain weight. We should look honestly at ourselves in the mirror. We can also use a belt and see whether or not we are now able to go "back" to the previous hole when on a weight loss program or remain using the same hole if trying to maintain our weight. We can also use a clothing item, such as a pair of trousers or a skirt, as a useful gauge. I have used the same skirt to keep my weight in check for over 15 years. It looks even better on me now than it did many years ago. Clothes will fit and look better as our bodies get leaner and more toned. In my opinion, this is a much more realistic check on our progress than scales.

We can also take an honest look at our faces and bodies. Our faces are usually a good indicator of whether we are losing or gaining weight. Take selfies or have our pictures taken. Are we happy with what we see?

We must understand that even if the figures on the scale are not to our liking, we will more than likely be making progress if we are eating and exercising mindfully. Let us start to focus more on the visual, as scales can drastically underrate or exaggerate our progress. Neither is good. The former can make us get discouraged and stop our weight loss/maintenance program, and the latter can give a false reality report which could be related purely to water loss only.

## Our Choice of Clothes

It is not a good idea to wear loose fitting clothes constantly over long periods. When we do, it is very easy to put on weight and not even know it for a while. I speak from my own experience here. I recall wearing loose fitting outfits over a sustained period. I was alarmed at the weight that had suddenly crept on me after I decided I wanted to wear a fitted outfit in my wardrobe. Clothes that are not loosely fitted help keep us in check. It reminds us when they start feeling snug that perhaps we need to watch our food intake and/or exercise more or differently. They can also help us to not overeat when we have them on during a meal.

This rule helped ensure that my weight remained stable through the 2020 Covid 19 lockdown that lasted for months. I often wore fitted clothes indoors to keep myself in check.

## Eating Out[21]

Eating in restaurants can be fun. It is probably a good idea though to consider eating out less and choose to cook more frequently at home with fresh ingredients. This way we have a much better idea of what we are eating.

While eating out, we should be aware of the ingredients that are often used in copious amounts to enhance the taste of foods in restaurants. Some of these can be greatly exaggerated and unexpected.

Small to moderate amounts of oil can have health benefits; however, restaurants generally use excessive amounts of oil for richer flavors, and these can make meals quite fattening.

## Butter

Butter is often used to make food taste richer. Many restaurants use copious amounts of this pure saturated fat in sauces, vegetables, etc. As we well know, we should be careful with saturated fats.

## Animal Fat

It is the streaks of animal fat in steaks when melted in cooking that gives a delicious and succulent flavor (as opposed to dry and tough) to a piece of meat. Unfortunately, too much of this saturated fat can be linked to high cholesterol levels.

## Salt

Restaurants often use salt to boost the flavor of their meals. Often too much is used. Salt is discussed more extensively in Chapter 5.

## Sweeteners

We expect added sugar in cakes and desserts. It is useful to know that sugar is often also used to enhance the flavor of bread, pasta, sauces, and vegetable, salad and other dressings.

## Portion Sizes

Most restaurants serve larger portion sizes than we actually need. Some also offer free sides like bread and butter. When eaten without care, they can cause us to consume more than our daily calories, carbs, and fat allocations before the main meal. Yikes!

## How to Improve Diet Quality?

To improve the overall quality of our diet, we must make sure most of our carbs, proteins, and fats are healthy. The nutrient dense variety is always best. The following check list will help get us there.

## Choose Whole Grains

When shopping for breads, cereals, and other grain-based foods, we should choose products with whole-grain ingredients listed first on the label. In main meals, replace some or all the white rice, pasta, or bread with brown rice, brown pasta, and quinoa.

## Cook and Eat Whole Foods

The best and highest-quality meals are based on minimally processed or unprocessed foods. Store-bought processed foods tend to pack in a lot of sugar, salt, fat, and additives such as food colorings and other enhancers. A sure-fire way to ensure healthy eating is to buy whole foods (vegetables, animal produce, fruits, and raw grains), and to prepare and cook them ourselves.

# Conclusion

I believe that if you have read this entire book, you will reach the same conclusion I have. Moderately eating ALL foods is unlikely to ensure weight loss. Rules are required. The most effective rule is eating moderate amounts of primarily, the nutrient dense foods that God has graciously blessed us with; in combination with exercise. This is the key to successful weight loss and maintenance.

Simply put it is not eating nutritious foods in moderation that ails us or causes weight gain. It is mindlessly eating overly processed foods that often causes havoc to our health.

The everyday choices we make to keep ourselves healthy are so important, both to our ability to do all God has planned for us, His purpose, and to the overall quality of our lives. Let us choose to live out our destiny intentionally by pursuing God's plan for our life. He already has it figured out. We just need to walk in it.[1] It matters to God what we do with our bodies. We should remember always that our bodies are His temple and so should be treated with respect.

Nobody else is responsible for our body: *we are.* For those who are married, your spouse is not responsible for looking after your body; ultimately you are. When faced with a spouse who lacks discipline and/or has eating habits that sabotage your efforts, you must dig deep and do what is best for you. Let's hope that with this determination we can be a positive influence.

We must learn to let the foods we put in our mouths do more to serve our future dreams and goals and less for our immediate unhealthy desires.[2] Let us strive to have a healthful, wholesome relationship with food. We must learn to make healthy choices and eat moderate amounts from these foods. We must not become slaves to what we eat.

Being intentional and mindful about how we eat and exercise today will help ensure that we live our best lives for all our tomorrows. The commitments we choose to make in life shape our life paths. If we look back over the years, we can probably recognize a handful of commitments that have determined where we are today.[3]

We all have a God-given, unique purpose. We must not let an ailing body get in the way or stop us from achieving God's unique purpose for our life. It is God's Will that we finish all that He planned for our life—His purpose.

When we decide to step away from unintentional living and its related frustrations, which include weight gain, various associated ailments, lethargy, disrupted sleep, etc.,[4] we give ourselves a good chance to achieve all God intended for us in every area of our lives.

Let's not be immoderate with our eating and exercise. If you are unable to say yes to God's plans, as a result of not eating and exercising mindfully, you will certainly not be experiencing fulfillment. Food for thought, right? God has entrusted you with your body, it's time to treat it well so that you can fully engage in your Creator's purpose for you.[5]

We must do our part to be healthy and trust God to bless our efforts.[6] He will bless us since He is ever faithful. A journey of a thousand steps begins with a single step.[7] Let us take moderate steps towards achieving a healthy lifestyle. A balanced approach has been proven to be the best way.

Moderation is key.

# Glossary of Terms

| Term | Definition |
|------|-----------|
| **Akara** | This is made with blended black-eyed beans. Seasonings, chopped onions, salt, tomatoes, pepper and some water are added to the beans mixture. Spoonfuls are then fried in hot vegetable oil. Akara is usually eaten at breakfast... |
| **Amstel** | A low sugar malt drink https://mobile.fatsecret.com/Diary.aspx? pa=fjrd&rid=2185015. June 2011. Accessed December 2018. |
| **Antioxidants** | These are chemical compounds that protect cells against the effects of free radicals. Free radicals are unstable atoms that can damage cells, causing illness and aging. There are a wide variety of foods with anti-oxidants. A few are berries, citrus fruits, nuts, carrots, spinach, parsley, onions, garlic and green tea. "Antioxidants: Why are they important?" https://www.mayoclinic.org/healthy-lifestyle/nutrition-and-healthy-eating/multimedia/antioxidants/sls-20076428. November 23, 2019. Accessed December 17, 2020. |
| **Beans** | These are black eyed beans. Their color (brownish) in Nigeria are different from the creamy color of the lookalike variety |

found in the US and many other countries. They have a similar taste though. They are boiled on their own or cooked in a tomato-based sauce. When boiled alone, they are often eaten as an accompaniment to boiled white rice, and/or with a stew and meat or fish.

**Beetroot**     This is the taproot portion of the beet plant. Beetroot is the term used in the U.K. In the U.S. it is referred to as beets. It is very nutritious with many health benefits, such as helping maintain a healthy weight, a good source of potassium and lowering blood pressure, to name a few.

Bjarnadottir, Adda. MS, RDN (Ice) "Beetroot 101: Nutrition Facts and Health Benefits."
https://www.healthline.com/nutrition/foods/beetroot.
March 8, 2019.Accessed December 2019.

**Biscuits**     These are about a quarter of an inch in thickness and usually sweet. They are primarily made from flour, butter and sugar, they can be plain or have various flavours and/ or creamy fillings. They are called biscuits in the U.K. and cookies in the U.S. In the U.S. biscuits look like the scones in the U.K., but, are not sweet.

**Chron's Disease**     This is a chronic inflammation of the bowel, that affects the lining of the digestive tract. This condition cannot be cured, but, it can be managed with anti-inflammatory medications such as steroids.

https://www.mayoclinic.org/diseases-conditions/crohns-disease/symptoms-causes/syc-20353304. October 13, 2020. Accessed December 17, 2020.

**Cocoyam**

This is a tropical root vegetable. It can be eaten boiled, roasted or fried.

It is high in fibre and contains complex carbohydrates that have a high GI, and so do not cause a spike in blood sugar. Its leaves are high in protein and are a good addition to some Nigerian soups.

"The Nutritional and Health Benefits of Cocoyam." https://www.pharmanewsonline.com/8216-2/. October 2016. Accessed December 17, 2020.

**Crisps**

These are typically made of very thinly sliced white/sweet potatoes that are deep fried. They are called crisps in the U.K. and chips in the U.S.

**Glycaemic Index**

This is the measurement of the relative ability of a carbohydrate food to increase the level of glucose in the blood. Foods with a low glycemic index (GI) release sugar into the blood at a slow rate. Conversely foods with a high GI can cause blood sugar to spike quite quickly on consumption. https://en.m.wikipedia.org/wiki/Glycemic_index. December 22, 2020. Accessed December 26, 2020.

**GMO Foods**

In the USA and some other countries,

food produce can be genetically altered. These products are labelled with the acronym for genetically modified organisms, GMO. These foods contain altered genetic material, using genetic engineering techniques. These foods can weaken our immunity, and are increasingly being found to be unhealthy in many other ways. Kennedy, Madeline and Cassetty, Samantha.

'Evidence-based pros and cons of GMO foods'

https://www.insider.com/gmo-pros-and-cons?amp

Nov 20, 2020. Accessed December 10, 2020.

**Guinea fowl**   This is a lean bird, popular in Africa. Its leanness makes it a healthier choice than chicken and beef. It has its own distinct flavour; some say a cross between turkey and quail.

http://www.grimaudfarms.com/fowl.htm. n.d. Accessed December 26, 2020.

**Moimoi**   This is a popular steamed bean pudding in Nigeria. The predominant ingredient is black-eyed beans as with akara above to which is added, onions, tomatoes, pepper, cray fish and other seasonings. The beans mixture for moimoi is more runny (thinner) than it is for akara. The beans mixture is best cooked poured and wrapped in leaves. It can also be cooked poured into plastic or foil containers. The parcels of the bean mixture and then steamed until they are cooked, 30-40 mins. It can be eaten at breakfast, on its own, with pap, or at other meals accompanied by rice and/or vegetables.

"How to Cook Nigerian Moi Moi with Leaves."https://www.allnigerianrecipes. com/howto/cook-moi-moi-leaves/. n.d. Accessed December 26, 2020.

**Nigerian vegetable soups**

These are typically tomato and onion-based soups that are well seasoned with ground crayfish, local spices and have various vegetables, meat and/or fish added to them.

**Ofada rice**

This is an unrefined, wild rice, with a very distinct smell popular in Nigeria. It is high in fibre, and contains lots of minerals and vitamins and is a healthy substitute for white rice.

**Pap**

This is made from dry white or yellow fermented corn. Pap has a distinct tangy sour taste, due to the fermentation process. It has the consistency of custard or grits. It can be eaten on its own or as an accompaniment to akara or moimoi. It is high in potassium and so helps to lower blood pressure. It is also a nutritious source of carbohydrates.

**Pepper soup**

This soup is popular in Nigeria. It is a broth-like soup made with hot peppers, various traditional spices, (some are medicinal) added. These soups can have various meats added, or can be made of only chicken, only fish etc. It is typically enjoyed as a starter, or when a light meal is desired and also enjoyed by many when not feeling very well. Just like many enjoy chicken soup when feeling poorly.

**Plantain**  This looks like a large banana and can be eaten unripe, when it is best eaten boiled or roasted. It is quite delicious eaten roasted, when it is half ripe. When ripe it is best eaten fried.

**Ribena**  This is usually a blackcurrant concentrate popular in the U.K. It has to be diluted, with plain or sparkling water before consumption.

**Squash drinks**  These are various fruit concentrates, that have to be diluted, usually with still water to taste before consumption. They are quite popular in the U.K.

**Stabilizing agent**  "What are Stabilizing Agents? What does FSSAI say?" https://foodsafetyhelpline.com/what-are-stabilizing-agents-what-does-fssai-say/?amp. October 12, 2015. Accessed December 2019.

**Swallow**  This is typically high in carbohydrates and can be made from a wide variety of carbohydrates, like, yam, plantain, ground rice, oatmeal, etc,
It is somewhat similar to mash potatoes, but not as fluffy...it is heavier. It is always accompanied by one of the many Nigerian soups.

**Sweet potatoes**  The species of this potato available is different depending on where you are in the world.
In West Africa, the variety available has a pinkish skin with a whitish flesh. In North America sweet potatoes have skin

with a more orangey color and the flesh is pinkish/orange in color

**Sweets**  These are called candy in the US.

**Thanksgiving**  This is a national holiday in the United States. It is celebrated on the fourth Thursday of November, with families and or/friends gathering to enjoy lots of food and making merry. A stuffed turkey is a staple in this feast, with many other delicious accompanying foods.

**Yam or sweet Potato pottage**  This is a one pot dish. The yam or sweet potatoes are cut into small pieces, bite size or slightly larger, and added and cooked in a sauce made up of onions, tomatoes, red peppers ground and sautéed in oil. Additional spices, salt, condiments and chopped green leaves are added which makes a delicious meal.

# ABOUT
# KHARIS PUBLISHING

**KHARIS PUBLISHING** is an independent, traditional publishing house with a core mission to publish impactful books, and channel proceeds into establishing mini-libraries or resource centers for orphanages in developing countries, so these kids will learn to read, dream, and grow. Every time you purchase a book from Kharis Publishing or partner as an author, you are helping give these kids an amazing opportunity to read, dream, and grow. Kharis Publishing is an imprint of Kharis Media LLC. Learn more at https://www.kharispublishing.com.

# CITED WORK

## Chapter 1

All references in this chapter, except for (2), are from devotional plans in the YouVersion Bible App online. They are typically book excerpts and are available for download using the Bible App.

[1] Searcy, Nelson and Dykes Henson, Jennifer. "The New You." YouVersion Devotional, Day 6. n.d. Accessed March 2019.

[2] Leaf, Caroline. "Think & Eat Yourself Smart." YouTube. https://youtu.be/Qo2mYL1Gh90. March 18, 2018. Accessed June 2019.

[3] Searcy, Nelson and Dykes Henson, Jennifer. "The New You." YouVersion Devotional, Day 3. n.d. Accessed March 2019.

[4] Stanley, Charles F. "Passion and Purpose." YouVersion Devotional, Day 5. n.d. Accessed January 2019.

[5] Evans, Tony. "Your purpose is in his hands." YouVersion Devotional, Day 1. n.d. Accessed July 2019.

[6] Stanley, Charles F. "Passion and Purpose." YouVersion Devotional, Day 5. n.d. Accessed January 2019.

[7] Searcy, Nelson and Dykes Henson, Jennifer. "The New You." YouVersion Devotional, Day 1. n.d. Accessed March 2019.

[8] Ibid.

[9] Ibid.

[10] Ibid. Day 2.

[11] Ibid. Day 3.

[12]Ibid. Day 2.

[13]Ibid.

[14]Ibid. Day 6.

[15]Ibid. Day 3.

[16]Ibid. Day 4.

## Chapter 2:

[1] "Fad diet."
Wikipedia https://en.m.wikipedia.org/wiki/Fad_diet. November17, 2020. Accessed December 4, 2020.

[2] Mawer, Rudy.
"The Ketogenic Diet: A Detailed Beginner's Guide to Keto."
https://www.healthline.com/nutrition/ketogenic-diet-101. October 22, 2020.

[3] Gordon, Barbara, RDN, LD.
"What is the Ketogenic Diet?"
https://www.eatright.org/health/weight-loss/fad-diets/what-is-the-ketogenic-diet
May 15, 2019. Reviewed April 2019. Accessed December 1, 2019.

[4] Lamotte, Sandee.
"Best diets' ranking puts keto last, DASH first."
https://amp.cnn.com/cnn/2018/01/04/health/keto-worst-diet-2018/index.html.
December 23, 2018. Accessed January 2019.

[5] Spritzler Franziska.
"The Dukan Diet Review: Does It Work for Weight Loss?"
https://www.healthline.com/nutrition/dukan-diet-101.
December 12, 2018. Accessed January 2019.

[6] iHerb staff writer.
"What is the Whole30 Diet?"
https://www.iherb.com/blog/what-is-the-whole30-di-

et/305?gclid=EAIaIQobChMIpdbClffS7QIVhNxRCh2O0gvW
EAAYASAAEgIWEPD_BwE&gclsrc=aw.ds. January 1, 2018.
Accessed January 2019.

[7] Gunnars, Kris, BSc.
"The Paleo Diet - A Beginner's Guide Plus Meal Plan."
healthline, https://www.healthline.com/nutrition/paleo-
diet-meal- plan-and-menu. August 1, 2018. Accessed January 2019.

[8] "12 Reasons To Stop Drinking Cow's Milk."
https://www.peta.org/living/food/reasons-stop-drinking-
milk/. June 27, 2019.
Accessed May 2020.

[9] "5 Common Food Sensitivities & Their Link to Autoimmune Diseases."
https://mindovermunch.com/blog/common-food-
sensitivities/. January 5, 2019. Accessed February 2019.

[10] Mayo Clinic Staff
"Mediterranean diet: A heart-healthy eating plan."
https://www.mayoclinic.org/healthy- lifestyle/nutrition-
and-healthy-eating/in-depth/mediterranean- diet/art-
20047801. June 21, 2019. Accessed August 2019.

[11]"DASH diet"
wikipedia, https://en.m.wikipedia.org/wiki/DASH_diet
October 21, 2020.Accessed December 17, 2020.

[12] Cherne, Kristeen.
Medically reviewed by Marengo, Katherine, LDN, R.D. "Can
the Keto Diet Cause Constipation?"
https://www.medicalnewstoday.com/articles/327040.
2019. Accessed January 2020.

[13] Lamotte, Sandee.
"Best diets' ranking puts keto last, DASH first."
https://amp.cnn.com/cnn/2018/01/04/health/keto-
worst-diet- 2018/index.html.
December 24, 2018. Accessed January 2019.

[14] Leaf, Caroline.
"Think & Eat Yourself Smart."
https://youtu.be/Qo2mYL1Gh90. 2018. Accessed June 2019.

[15]Ibid.

## Chapter 3:

[1] National Institutes of Health. "Nutrient-dense food." https:// ww.cancer.gov/publications/dictionaries/cancer-terms/def/nutrient-dense-food. n.d. Accessed December 18, 2020.

[2] Harvard Health Publishing. "Add more nutrient-dense foods to your diet." https://www.health.harvard.edu/staying- healthy/add-more-nutrient-dense-foods-to-your-diet. July 2015. Accessed October 2018.

[3] Leaf, Caroline. "Think & Eat Yourself Smart." YouTube. https://youtu.be/Qo2mYL1Gh90. 2018. Accessed June 2019.

[4] Cleveland Clinic medical professional. "Carbohydrates." https://my.clevelandclinic.org/health/articles/15416-carbohydrates. March 15, 2014. Accessed October 2018.

[5] JohJohnson, Olivia.
"The Fundamentals of a Balanced Diet: Foods, Benefits, Weight Loss." https://betterme.world/articles/balanced-diet/?utm_source=google&utm_medium=cpc&utm_campaign=recur-ring_chinese_s/221&utm_content=482599562562&utm_term=&gclid=EAIaIQobChMIyKen3OTU7QIVumDmCh0bQgwgEAAYASA AEgJ6O_D_BwE. 2020. Accessed December 18, 2020.

[6] Harvard Health Publishing. "Carbohydrates in your diet: It's the quality that counts."

https://www.health.harvard.edu/mens-health/carbohydrates-in-your-diet-its-the-quality-that-counts. February 2014. Accessed October 3, 2020.

[7] Wikipedia. "Protein (nutrient)." https://en.m.wikipedia.org/wiki/Protein_(nutrient). December 8, 2020.
Accessed December 18, 2020.

[8]Cedars-Sinai staff "Are Animal Proteins Better for You Than Plant Proteins?"

https://www.cedars-sinai.org/blog/best-protein.html. Jan 16, 2019. Accessed February 2019.

[9] Leaf, Caroline. "Think & Eat Yourself Smart." YouTube. https://youtu.be/Qo2mYL1Gh90. 2018. Accessed June 2019.

[10] Gunnars,Kris"10 Science-Backed Reasons to Eat More Protein." https://www.healthline.com/nutrition/10-reasons-to-eat-more-protein#TOC_TITLE_HDR_2
March 8, 2019. Accessed April, 2019.

[11]"Protein." https://www.betterhealth.vic.gov.au/health/healthyliving/protein. n.d. Accessed December 18, 2020.

[12] Leaf, Caroline.
"Think & Eat Yourself Smart."
YouTube, https://youtu.be/Qo2mYL1Gh90
2018.
Accessed June, 2019

[13] National Health Service. "Fish and shellfish - Eat well." https://www.nhs.uk/live-well/eat-well/fish-and-shellfish-nutrition/.
December 4, 2018. Accessed January 2019.

[14] Leech, Joe. MS "Legumes: Good or Bad?"healthline, https://www.healthline.com/nutrition/legumes-good-or-badJuly 29, 2019. Accessed August 2019.

[15] "Nuts and seeds."
https://www.betterhealth.vic.gov.au/health/healthyliving/Nuts-and-seeds
October 31, 2012
Accessed December, 2018.

[16] Robinson, Lawrence., Segal, Jeanne. Ph.D., and Segal, Robert. M.A. "Choosing Healthy Fats."
https://www.helpguide.org/articles/healthy-eating/choosing-healthy-fats.htm
December 17, 2020

[17] "Potential Health Benefits of Plant v. Marine Omega-3 Fatty Acids."
http://med.stanford.edu/nutrition/nutrition-studies-group/completed-studies/plant-vs-marine-omega-3s.html
Accessed December 18, 2020

[18] "When it Comes to Fat, How Hot is Too Hot?"
https://www.marksdailyapple.com/oil-fat-overheat-smoking-point/
September 10, 2020
December 16, 2020

[19] Leaf, Caroline.
"Think & Eat Yourself Smart." YouTube,
https://youtu.be/Qo2mYL1Gh90
2018
Accessed June 2019

[20] Ibid.

[21] Ibid.

[22] Ibid.

## Chapter 4:

[1] Wikipedia. "Yo-yo effect."
https://en.m.wikipedia.org/wiki/Yo-yo_effect.   September 23, 2020. Accessed December 4, 2020.

[2] "Defeating Emotional Cravings and Temptation."
equalition, https://equalution.com/blogs/news/defeating-emotional-cravings-and-temptation
Accessed December 18, 2020

[3] Moss, Michael. Reviewed by Blythman, Joanna.
"Salt Sugar Fat: How the Food Giants Hooked Us."
https://amp.theguardian.com/books/2013/feb/24/salt-sugar-fat-moss-review
24 Feb 2013. Accessed April 2019

[4] "Carbohydrates in your diet: It's the quality that counts."
https://www.health.harvard.edu/mens-health/carbohydrates-in-your-diet-its-the-quality-that-counts
February, 2014.
Accessed October 3, 2020

[5] "9 Foods You Can Eat at Night Without Gaining..."
Youtube. https://youtu.be/H-fcwL3rkm8
2018. Accessed February, 2019

[6] Caroline Leaf. "Think & Eat Yourself Smart."
YouTube, https://youtu.be/Qo2mYL1Gh90
2018. Accessed June 2019.

[7] Nadeem, Maria. "Mindful eating verses mindless eating."
https://medcraveonline.com/AOWMC/mindful-eating-verses-mindless-eating.html
Published March 16, 2016.
Accessed December 4, 2020

[8] "Here's What Happens When You Eat Too Much."
https://www.tesh.com/articles/here-s-what-happens-when-you-eat-too-much/
December. 1, 2016.
Accessed Dec. 2018

[9] Leaf, Caroline. "Think & Eat Yourself Smart."
YouTube, https://youtu.be/Qo2mYL1Gh90
2018. Accessed June 2019

10 (i)   "How the French stay so slim."
YouTube, https://youtu.be/mEecd9bPYxc
2015. Accessed December, 2018.

(ii) "How The French Eat." YouTube.
https://youtu.be/oKpW6J1LNyU. 2020.
Accessed December 17, 2020.

(iii) "Why are French women so thin & the food so good."
YouTube. https://youtu.be/RRB4nlFo4XA. 2017. Accessed
December 2018.

11 Godsey, Cynthia, Horowitz, Diane, MD, Sather, Rita, RN.
"Garlic."
https://www.urmc.rochester.edu/encyclopedia/content.a
spx?contenttypeid=19&contentid=Garlic
Accessed December 18, 2020

12 "nutrient-dense food."
https://www.cancer.gov/publications/dictionaries/cancer
-terms/def/nutrient-dense-food
Accessed December 16,2020

## Chapter 5:

1 Moss, Michael. Reviewed by Joanna Blythman.
"Salt Sugar Fat: How the Food Giants Hooked Us."
https://amp.theguardian.com/books/2013/feb/24/salt-
sugar-fat-moss-review
February 24, 2013. Accessed April 2019.

2 Scutti, Susan. "Overprocessed foods add 500 calories to
your diet every day, causing weight gain."
https://amp.cnn.com/cnn/2019/05/17/health/ultraproc
essed-foods-weight-gain-study-trnd/index.html
May 17, 2019. Accessed December 2020.

3 (i) Armstrong, Eric. "What's Wrong with High Fructose
Corn Syrup?"
https://treelight.com/health/nutrition/whats-wrong-
with-high-fructose-corn-syrup/
April, 2017. Accessed June 2019.

(ii)Cherney Kristeen.
Medically reviewed by Butler, Natalie. R.D., L.D.
Healthline, "5 Ways to Avoid Hydrogenated Oil"
https://www.healthline.com/health/ways-to-avoid-hydrogenated-oil
September 28, 2018. Accessed December 17, 2020.

(iii) Leaf, Caroline. "Think & Eat Yourself Smart." YouTube.
https://youtu.be/Qo2mYL1Gh90. 2018. Accessed June 2019.

4 Elliott, Brianna. RD. "20 Foods With High-Fructose Corn Syrup."
https://www.healthline.com/nutrition/20-foods-with-high-fructose-corn-syrup
November 10, 2016.
Accessed June 2019.

5 Parker, Hilary. Princeton University Science Daily. "High-Fructose Corn Syrup Prompts Considerably More Weight Gain, researchers find."
https://www.sciencedaily.com/releases/2010/03/10032 2121115.htm?utm_source=feedburner&utm_medium=fee d&utm_campaign=Feed%3A+sciencedaily+%28ScienceDai ly%3A+Latest+Science+N ews%29.
March 22, 2010. Accessed June 2019.

6 Mayo Clinic Staff.
"Metabolic Syndrome."
https://www.mayoclinic.org/diseases-conditions/metabolic-syndrome/symptoms-causes/syc-20351916
March 14, 2019.
Accessed June 2019

7 Link, Rachael, MS, RD Medically reviewed by Bjarnadot-tir, Adda. MS, RDN. "What Is Hydrogenated Vegetable Oil?"
https://www.healthline.com/nutrition/hydrogenated-vegetable-oil
September 25, 2019. Accessed October 3, 2019.

[8] "Trans fat is double trouble for your heart health."
https://www.mayoclinic.org/diseases-conditions/high-blood-cholesterol/in-depth/trans-fat/art-20046114
Feb. 13, 2020. Accessed October 3, 2020.

[9] Wikipedia. "Trans fat regulation."
https://en.m.wikipedia.org/wiki/Trans_fat_regulation
December 14, 2020. Accessed December 19, 2020.

[10] Belluz, Julia and Collins, Dylan. "The new global plan to eliminate the most harmful fat in food, explained."
https://www.vox.com/platform/amp/science-and-health/2018/5/14/17346108/trans-fats-food-world-health-organization-bloomberg-gates
May 14, 2018. Accessed October 3, 2019.

[11] Hosmer, Caitlin. M.S., R.D. "Does "no trans fat" really mean no trans fat?"
https://www.health.harvard.edu/newsletter_article/ask-the-doctor-does-no-trans-fat-really-mean-no-trans-fat
October 2006. Accessed October 3, 2019.

[12] "Trans fat is double trouble for your heart health."
https://www.mayoclinic.org/diseases-conditions/high-blood-cholesterol/in-depth/trans-fat/art-20046114
February 13, 2020. Accessed May 23, 2020.

[13] Proodian, James, Dr. "Natural healthcare Center Article - Why Trans Fats and High- Fructose Corn Syrup Must Be Banned." https://naturalhealthcarecenter.com/why-trans-fats-and-high- fructose-corn-syrup-must-be-banned/.
March 12, 2014. Accessed October 3, 2019.

[14] Leaf, Caroline. "Think & Eat Yourself Smart."
YouTube. https://youtu.be/Qo2mYL1Gh90
2018. Accessed June 2019

[15] Wikipedia. "Food processing."
https://en.m.wikipedia.org/wiki/Food_processing
November 30, 2020
Accessed December 17, 2020

16 Chan, T. H. "Processed Foods and Health."
https://www.hsph.harvard.edu/nutritionsource/processed-foods/
June 24, 2019. Accessed December 23, 2020

17 Leaf, Caroline. "Think & Eat Yourself Smart."
YouTube.https://youtu.be/Qo2mYL1Gh90 2018.
Accessed June 2019.

18 "Trans fat is double trouble for your heart health."
https://www.mayoclinic.org/diseases-conditions/high-blood-cholesterol/in-depth/trans-fat/art-20046114
February 13, 2020. Accessed May 23, 2020.

19 Myers, Dan. "5 Things You Didn't Know About Wonder Bread." https://abcnews.go.com/amp/Lifestyle/things-didnt-bread/story?id=29424069. March 6, 2015. December 2019.

20 Moss, Michael. Reviewed by Joanna Blythman.
"Salt Sugar Fat: How the Food Giants Hooked Us."
https://amp.theguardian.com/books/2013/feb/24/salt-sugar-fat-moss-review February 24, 2013. Accessed April 2019.

21 Leaf, Caroline. "Think & Eat Yourself Smart."
YouTube, https://youtu.be/Qo2mYL1Gh90. 2018
Accessed June 2019.

22 Wikipedia. "Convenience food."
https://en.m.wikipedia.org/wiki/Convenience_food.
December 8, 2020. Accessed December 23, 2020.

23 Leaf, Caroline. "Think & Eat Yourself Smart." YouTube.
https://youtu.be/Qo2mYL1Gh90. 2018. Accessed June 2019.

24 Ibid.

25 "Fuel for your body."
http://www.cyh.com/healthtopics/library/fuel_for_your_body.pdf. February 2011.
Accessed January2019

[26] Leaf, Caroline. "Think & Eat Yourself Smart." YouTube. https://youtu.be/Qo2mYL1Gh90. 2018. Accessed June 2019.

[27] The Ellen Degeneres Show. "Charlize Theron ate potato chips to gain weight for "Tully"."
YouTube. https://youtu.be/pK0_gE8hRCM. 2018 Accessed March 2019.

[28] Zeratsky, Katherine, R.D., L.D. "Junk food blues: Are depression and diet related?"
https://www.mayoclinic.org/diseases- conditions/depression/expert-answers/depression-and-diet/faq- 20058241. February 10, 2018. Accessed March 2019.

[29] Avramova, Nina. "A small glass of juice or soda a day is linked to increased risk of cancer, study finds."
https://amp.cnn.com/cnn/2019/07/10/health/sugary-drinks- cancer-risk-study-intl/index.html. July 12, 2019. Accessed July 2, 2020.

[30] Dumain, Theresa. "10 Tricks to Cut Out Sugar andImprove Arthritis Symptoms (and Not Even Miss It)."
https://creakyjoints.org/diet-exercise/eat-less-sugar-manage-arthritis/. December, 2018. Accessed March 2019

[31] "Six Keys to Reducing Inflammation."
https://www.scripps.org/news_items/4232-six-keys-to-reducing-inflammation.
January 15, 2020. Accessed December 17, 2020.

[32] Brown, Mary Jane, PhD, RD. "Does Sugar Cause Inflammation in the Body?"
(Point 37). https://www.healthline.com/nutrition/sugar-and- inflammation.
November 12, 2017. Accessed May 6, 2018.

[33] Miller, Julie. "Does Diet Soda Cause Sweet Cravings?"
healthfully, https://healthfully.com/517129-does-diet-soda-cause- sweet-cravings.html. August 23, 2011. Accessed December 29, 2020.

[34] West, Helen, RD. "Do Artificial Sweeteners Harm Your Good Gut Bacteria?" https://www.healthline.com/nutrition/artificial-
sweeteners-and-gut-bacteria.
September 13, 2017. Accessed December 2019.

[35] LaMotte, Sandee. "Drinking two or more diet beverages a day linked to high risk of stroke, heart attacks."
https://amp.cnn.com/cnn/2019/02/14/health/diet-soda-
women-stroke-heart-attack/index.html. February 16, 2019. Accessed March 2019.

## Chapter 6:

[1] Bellisle, France, Dr. "The Factors That Influence Our Food Choices." INRA, France.

https://www.eufic.org/en/healthy-living/article/the-   de-
terminants-of-food-choice. June 2006. Accessed January 2019.

[2] Axe, Josh, Dr. "The Daniel diet-How to do the Daniel Fast." YouTube.
https://youtu.be/xV5mm0zwvtc. 2015. Accessed February 2019.

[3] Brown, Mary Jane   PhD, RD (UK) — Medically reviewed by Arnarson, Atli. BSc, PhD. Juicing: Good or bad?
https://www.healthline.com/nutrition/juicing-good-or-
bad. October 4, 2019. Accessed November 2019

[4] Tavernise, Sabrina. "Fancy Juice Doesn't Cleanse the Body of Toxins."
https://www.nytimes.com/2016/04/21/health/juice-
cleanse-toxin-misconception.amp.html.   April   20,   2016.
Accessed February 2019.

[5] "Grapefruit Juice and Some Drugs Don't Mix."
https://www.fda.gov/consumers/consumer-
updates/grapefruit-juice-and-some-drugs-dont-mix
July 18, 2017. Accessed March, 2019.

[6] (i) Corona, Natalie. "How to start intermittent fasting for beginners." YouTube. https://youtu.be/ElIgUgK-ZM0. 2018. Accessed March 2019.

(ii) Whittel, Naomi. "The Ultimate Guide to Intermittent Fasting." YouTube. https://youtu.be/T78vPC7g1jc. 2019. Accessed March 2020.

(iii) Thurlow, Cynthia. "Intermittent Fasting: Transformational Technique." Ted Talk. YouTube. https://youtu.be/A6Dkt7zyImk. 2019. Accessed March 2020.

## Chapter 7:

[1] Belluz, Julia. "Most of us misunderstand metabolism. Here are 9 facts to clear that up." https://www.vox.com/platform/amp/2016/5/18/11685254/metabolism-definition-booster-weight-loss. September 4, 2018. Accessed April 2019

[2] West, Helen, RD. "10 Easy Ways to Boost Your Metabolism (Backed by Science)." https://www.healthline.com/nutrition/10-ways-to- boost-metabolism#TOC_TITLE_HDR_1. July 27, 2018. Accessed December 2019.

[3] Ibid.

[4] Ibid.

[5] Ibid.

[6] Ibid.

[7] Belluz, Julia. "Most of us misunderstand metabolism. Here are 9 facts to clear that up." https://www.vox.com/platform/amp/2016/5/18/11685254/metabolism-definition-booster-weight-loss.September 4, 2018. Accessed April 2019.

[8] Jacques, Jacqueline, ND. "The Role of Your Thyroid in Metabolism and Weight Control."

https://www.obesityaction.org/community/article-library/the-role-of-your-thyroid-in-metabolism-and-weight-control/.Winter 2009. Accessed December 2019.

## Chapter 8:

[1] Blair, Steven N. "Exercise." https://www.britannica.com/topic/exercise-physical-fitness. November 20, 2020. Accessed November 25, 2020.

[2] Armstrong, Dixon, et al. "Physical inactivity." https://www.who.int/publications/cra/chapters/volume 1/0729- 0882.pdf. n.d. Accessed December 19, 2020.

[3] Blair, Steven N. "Exercise." https://www.britannica.com/topic/exercise-physical-fitness November 20, 2020. Accessed November 25, 2020

[4] Laskowski, Edward R. "How much should the average adult exercise every day?" https://www.mayoclinic.org/healthy-lifestyle/fitness/expert-answers/exercise/faq-20057916 April 27, 2019. Accessed December 1, 2020

[5] Chertoff, Jane. Medically reviewed by Daniel Bubnis, M.S., NASM-CPT, NASE Level II-CSS. "What's the Difference Between Aerobic and Anaerobic?" https://www.healthline.com/health/fitness- exercise/difference-between-aerobic-and-anaerobic. September 1, 2018. Accessed October 2018.

[6] "How the French stay so slim." YouTube. https://youtu.be/mEecd9bPYxc. 2015. Accessed October 2018.

[7] Searcy, Nelson and Dykes Henson, Jennifer. "The New You." YouVersion Devotional, Day 3. n.d. Accessed March 2019.

[8] Cafasso, Jacquelyn. Medically reviewed by Sampson, Stacy, D.O. "Why Do We Need Endorphins?"

https://www.healthline.com/health/endorphins. July 11, 2017. Accessed December 2018.

[9] Searcy, Nelson and Dykes Henson, Jennifer. "The New You." YouVersion Devotional, Day 2. n.d. Accessed March 2019.

[10] Tinsley, Grant. PhD. "Should You Eat Before or After Working Out?" https://www.healthline.com/nutrition/eating-before-or-after-workout. May 27, 2018. Accessed December, 2018

[11]Lindberg, Sara. Medically reviewed by Deborah Weatherspoon, Ph.D., R.N., CRNA. "Can You Lose Weight Faster by Exercising on an Empty Stomach?" https://www.healthline.com/health/fitness-exercise/fasted-cardio-when-to-eat-workout. September 11, 2018. Accessed December, 2018.

[12] Harvey-Jenner, Catriona. "This is what will happen to your body if you don't eat after a workout. Basically: eat." cosmopolitan, https://cosmomag.lk/tag/muscles/ October 24, 2017. Accessed December 2018

[13]Mischel, Fiona. Medically reviewed by Melinda Maryniuk, MEd, RDN, CDE, FADA. "10 Symptoms of Low Blood Sugar After Exercise." https://www.livestrong.com/article/102754-low-blood-sugar-symptoms-after/. November 26, 2019. Accessed December 2019.

[14] Bergeson Becco, Laine. FMCHC. "How Exercise Affects Circulation (and Vice Versa)" https://experiencelife.com/article/how-exercise-affects-circulation-and-vice-versa/amp/ Accessed December 19, 2020.

## Chapter 9:

[1] (i) Terrell, Casey, MPH, RD. "Food Allergy or Intolerance: What's the Difference?" https://foodinsight.org/food-allergy-or-intolerance-whats-the-difference/?gclid=EAIaIQobChMIxPKTnJra7QIVFWHmCh3XMgMYEAAY ASAAEgJ0J_D_BwE. May 16, 2019. Accessed December 2019.

(ii) "Food allergy and intolerance." https://www.betterhealth.vic.gov.au/health/conditionsandtreatments/food-allergy-and-intolerance. July 31, 2013. Accessed December 2019.

[2]Wikipedia. "Gluten." https://en.m.wikipedia.org/wiki/Gluten. December 12, 2020. Accessed December 19, 2020.

[3] Leaf, Caroline. "Think and eat yourself smart." YouTube, https://youtu.be/Qo2mYL1Gh90.2018 Accessed June 2019.

[4] Bjarnadottir, Adda. MS, RDN (Ice). "The 14 Most Common Signs of Gluten Intolerance." https://www.healthline.com/nutrition/signs-you-are-gluten-intolerant.September 29, 2016. Accessed April 2019

[5] "Celiac Disease." https://www.mayoclinic.org/diseases-conditions/celiac-disease/symptoms-causes/syc-20352220 October 21, 2020. Accessed November 4, 2020

[6] Fletcher, Jenna. Medically reviewed by Elaine K. Luo, M.D. "What happens in gluten ataxia?" https://www.medicalnewstoday.com/articles/320730. January 25, 2018. Accessed February 2019.

[7] "Lactose intolerance." https://www.mayoclinic.org/diseases-conditions/lactose-intolerance/symptoms-causes/syc-20374232 April 07, 2020. Accessed November 21, 2020

[8] "Inflammatory Bowel Disease Clinic."

http://www.ibdclinic.ca/ibd-and-lifestyle/ibd-and-diet/lactose-intolerance/. Accessed December 26, 2020

[9] "Peanut, Tree Nut and Seed Allergy." https://www.allergy.org.au/patients/food-allergy/peanut-tree-nut-and-seed-allergy. May 2019. Accessed June 2019

[10] Burgess, Sanya. "Mum of Pret allergy victim Natasha Ednan-Laperouse weeps at inquest after hearing defibrillator was not used in-flight."
sky news, https://news.sky.com/story/amp/mother-of-pret-allergy-victim-weeps-at-inquest-after-defibrillator-was-not-used-in-flight-11509377
27 September 2018. Accessed June 2019

[11] "Shellfish allergy." https://www.mayoclinic.org/diseases-conditions/shellfish-allergy/symptoms-causes/syc-20377503
June 19, 2020. Accessed November 21, 2020

[12] "Peanut, Tree Nut and Seed Allergy." https://www.allergy.org.au/patients/food-allergy/peanut-tree-nut-and-seed-allergy
Updated May 2019. Accessed June 2019

## Chapter 10:

[1] Leech, Joe, MS. Medically reviewed by, Atli Arnarson, BSc, PhD."10 reasons why good sleep is important." https://www.healthline.com/nutrition/10-reasons-why-good-sleep-is-important. n.d. Accessed December 19, 2020.

[2] Taheri, Lin, et al. "Short Sleep Duration Is Associated with Reduced Leptin, Elevated Ghrelin, and Increased Body Mass Index." Abstract. PLoS medicine. https://www.ncbi.nlm.nih.gov/pmc/articles/PMC535701/. December 2004. Accessed December 21, 2020.

[3](i) "Getting past a weight-loss plateau."
https://www.mayoclinic.org/healthy-lifestyle/weight-loss/in-depth/weight-loss-plateau/art-20044615.  February 25, 2020. Accessed December 17, 2020.

(ii) Spritzler, Franziska. "14 Simple Ways to Break Through a Weight Loss Plateau."
https://www.healthline.com/nutrition/weight-loss-plateau#TOC_TITLE_HDR_2. February 27, 2017. Accessed August 23, 2020.

[4]Dansinger, Michael. MD. "Insulin Resistance."
https://www.webmd.com/diabetes/insulin-resistance-syndrome.
July 1, 2019. Accessed December 2, 2019.

[5] Roland, James. "Signs of Insulin Resistance."
https://www.healthline.com/health/diabetes/insulin-resistance-symptoms#TOC_TITLE_HDR_1
September 2, 2014. Accessed September 2019

[6] "What is 'gut health' and why is it important?"
https://health.ucdavis.edu/health-news/newsroom/what-is-gut-health-and-why-is-it-important/2019/07
July 22, 2019. October 6, 2020

[7]Parent Walravens, Samantha. "10 signs You Have a Leaky Gut..."
https://www.healthywomen.org/amp/10-signs-you-have-leaky-gutand-how-heal-it-2646337605.
November 26, 2013. Accessed November 15, 2020.

[8] Frothingham,Scott Medically reviewed by Sethi, Saurabh, M.D., MPH. "How Long Does It Take to Heal a Leaky Gut?"
https://www.healthline.com/health/how-long-does-it-take-to-heal-leaky-gut#causes
September 4, 2019. Accessed November 15, 2020

[9] "Cushing Syndrome."

https://www.mayoclinic.org/diseases-conditions/cushing-syndrome/symptoms-causes/syc-20351310
May 30, 2019. December 2019

[10] Bergland, Christopher.
"Cortisol: Why the "Stress Hormone" Is Public Enemy No. 1."
https://www.psychologytoday.com/us/blog/the-athletes-way/201301/cortisol-why-the-stress-hormone-is-public-enemy-no-1?amp. Jan 22, 2013. Accessed February 12, 2019

[11] De Pietro, MaryAnn. CRT. Medically reviewed by Ranchod, Yamini. Ph.D., M.S. "What are the benefits and risks of a sauna?"
https://www.medicalnewstoday.com/articles/313109
June 17, 2019. Accessed September 2019

[12] "Slideshow: Thyroid Symptoms and Solutions."
https://www.webmd.com/women/ss/slideshow-thyroid-symptoms-and-solutions
Accessed December 17, 2020.

[13] "Can I Blame My Weight on My Thyroid?"
https://www.premierhealth.com/your-health/articles/women-wisdom-wellness-/can-i-blame-my-weight-on-my-thyroid-. Mar 13, 2017. Accessed September 2019

[14] Shomon, Mary. Medically reviewed by Waldman, Lindsey. MD, RD. "Diet and Weight Loss Tips for Thyroid Patients."
https://www.verywellhealth.com/diet-and-weight-loss-tips-for-thyroid-patients-3233060
November 06, 2019. Accessed December 13, 2019

[15] "Hypothyroidism (underactive thyroid)."
https://www.mayoclinic.org/diseases-conditions/hypothyroidism/symptoms-causes/syc-20350284

November. 19, 2020. Accessed December 3, 2020

[16] Raman, Ryan. MS, RD Medically reviewed by Arnarson, Atli. BSc, PhD. "Best Diet for Hypothyroidism: Foods to Eat, Foods to Avoid." https://www.healthline.com/nutrition/hypothyroidism-diet. November 15, 2019. Accessed December 13, 2019

[17] "Obesity and hormones." https://www.betterhealth.vic.gov.au/health/healthyliving/obesity-and-hormones Accessed December 18, 2020.

[18] Gotter, Ana. Medically reviewed by Bubnis, Daniel. M.S., NASM-CPT, NASE Level II-CSS. "How is visceral fat rated and measured?" https://www.healthline.com/health/visceral-fat#rating-and-measurements. September 17, 2018. Accessed June 2019

[19] T.H. Chan. "Genes Are Not Destiny." https://www.hsph.harvard.edu/obesity-prevention-source/obesity-causes/genes-and-obesity/ April 11, 2016. Accessed June 2019.

## Chapter 11:

[1] Leaf, Caroline. "Think & Eat Yourself Smart." YouTube. https://youtu.be/Qo2mYL1Gh90. 2018. Accessed June 2019.

[2] Searcy, Nelson, and Dykes Henson, Jennifer. "The New You." YouVersion Devotional, Day 4. n.d. Accessed March 2019.

[3] Searcy, Nelson, and Dykes Henson, Jennifer. "The New You." YouVersion Devotional, Day 6. n.d. Accessed March 2019.

[4]Searcy, Nelson, and Dykes Henson, Jennifer. "The New You." YouVersion Devotional, Day 4. n.d. Accessed March 2019.

[5]Searcy, Nelson, and Dykes Henson, Jennifer. "The New You." YouVersion Devotional, Day 2. n.d. Accessed March 2019.

[6] Langford, Eliizabeth. "Are you a Closet Eater? 4 Ways to Curb the Binge." https://www.natalieshay.com/blogs/are-you-a-closet-eater-4-ways-to-curb-the-binge?format=amp May 28, 2018. Accessed November 2019

[7]Searcy, Nelson, and Dykes Henson, Jennifer. "The New You." YouVersion Devotional, Day 7.n.d. Accessed March 2019.

[8]Ibid.

[9]Ibid.

[10]Ibid.

[11]Searcy, Nelson, and Dykes Henson, Jennifer. "The New You." YouVersion Devotional, Day 5. n.d. Accessed March 2019.

[12]Ibid.

[13]Ibid.

## Chapter 12:

[1] "Stress." https://my.clevelandclinic.org/health/articles/11874-stress. May 2, 2015. Accessed July 2019.

[2] "Stress and your health." https://medlineplus.gov/ency/article/003211.htm October 5, 2020. Accessed December 17, 2020

[3] "Shingles." https://www.mayoclinic.org/diseases- conditions/shingles/symptoms-causes/syc-20353054. October 6, 2020. Accessed December 17, 2020.

[4] Ware, Megan, RDN, L.D. Medically reviewed by Debra Sullivan, Ph.D., MSN, R.N., CNE, COI."What are the health benefits of vitamin D?"
https://www.medicalnewstoday.com/articles/161618. November 7, 2019. Accessed September 17, 2020.

[5] Yao,Song. et *al.*
"Associations between vitamin D deficiency and risk of aggressive breast cancer in African-American women." Abstract. https://pubmed.ncbi.nlm.nih.gov/22995734/. July 2013. Accessed July 2019.

[6]Hess, Julie M., Jonnalagadda, Satya S., Slavin, Joanne L. "What Is a Snack, Why Do We Snack, and How Can We Choose Better Snacks? A Review of the Definitions of Snacking, Motivations to Snack, Contributions to Dietary Intake, and Recommendations for Improvement." https://academic.oup.com/advances/article/7/3/466/45 58044? login=true.
May 9, 2016. Accessed July 2019.

[7] Leonard, Jayne. Medically reviewed by Butler, Natalie. R.D., L.D. "Is honey better for you than sugar?"
https://www.medicalnewstoday.com/articles/317728#_n oHeaderPrefixedContent
June 1, 2017. July 2019

[8] (I)) Hill, Ansley. RD, LD. "Should You Have Cheat Meals or Cheat Days?"
https://www.healthline.com/nutrition/cheat-meals September 13, 2019. Accessed December 2019

(ii) Fitzpatrick, Kelly and Lebow, Hilary. Medically reviewed by Hatanaka, Miho, RDN, L.D.
"Are Cheat Meals Bad for You? Cheat Days Explained." https://greatist.com/health/cheat-days-explained September 3, 2019. Accessed December 2019

[9] Maynard, Andrea Quigley. "A Better Relationship with Food Means Making Deliberate Decisions." https://aqmhealthcoaching.com/2016/12/01/a-better-relationship-with-food-means-making-deliberate-decisions/amp/ 2016. Accessed December 2019

[10] Farooqi, Sadaf. The Intelligence Podcast. University of Cambridge Research on obesity. 31Peter Wilson, for 1843, The Economist sister magazine. Excerpts from discussion on calories. Discussion on calories is at about 17 mins from the beginning of the podcast. "Unbalance of trade: China-America talks." https://itunes.apple.com/WebObjects/MZStore.woa/wa/viewPodcast?id=291942390#episodeGuid=8bfe3662-464b-4341-af9e-021e4a06c83d May 10, 2019, Accessed May 14, 2019.

[11] Nguyen, P K., Lin, S., and Heidenreich, P. "A systematic comparison of sugar content in low-fat vs regular versions of food." Abstract. https://www.ncbi.nlm.nih.gov/pmc/articles/PMC4742721/ November, 2015. Accessed December 2019.

[12] University of Arkansas. "Most Consumers Misinterpret Meaning of Trans-Fat Information on Nutrition Facts Panel, Study Shows." https://phys.org/news/2008-06-consumers-misinterpret-trans-fat-nutrition-facts.amp June 18, 2008. Accessed December 2019.

[13]Bjarnadottir, Adda, MS, RDN (Ice). Medically reviewed by Kathy W. Warwick, R.D., CDE. "The 56 Most Common Names for Sugar (Some Are Tricky)." https://www.healthline.com/nutrition/56-different-names-for-sugar June 26, 2020. Accessed December 17, 2020.

[14] Leaf, Caroline. "Think and eat yourself smart." YouTube, https://youtu.be/Qo2mYL1Gh90 Uploaded 2018. Accessed June 2019.

[15] Ibid.

16 Brett Parnes, Robin. "Why is Organic Food So Expensive?"
https://science.howstuffworks.com/environmental/green
- science/organic-food6.htm. January 27, 2020. Accessed March 2020.

17 Leaf, Caroline. "Think and eat yourself smart."
YouTube, https://youtu.be/Qo2mYL1Gh90. 2018
Accessed June 2019.

18 Ibid.

19 Ibid.

20 Davies, Jeanie Lerche. "Bathroom Scales Don't Tell The Whole Story."
https://www.webmd.com/diet/obesity/features/body-fat- measurements. June 9, 2005. Accessed June 2019.

21 Smith, Holly. "What regularly dining out does to your body."
https://www.insider.com/what-dining-out-does-to-your-body-2018-6?amp June 2018. Accessed June 2019.

## Conclusion:

1 Evans, Tony. "Your purpose is in his hands." YouVersion Devotional, Day 1. n.d. Accessed July 2019.

2 Searcy, Nelson and Dykes Henson, Jennifer. "The New You." YouVersion Devotional -, Day 5 n.d. Accessed March 2019.

3 Searcy, Nelson and Dykes Henson, Jennifer. "The New You." YouVersion Devotional, Day 2. n.d. Accessed March 2019.

4 Ibid.

5 Searcy, Nelson and Dykes Henson, Jennifer. "The New You." YouVersion Devotional, Day 1. n.d. Accessed March 2019.

[6] Searcy, Nelson and Dykes Henson, Jennifer. "The New You." YouVersion Devotional, Day 2. n.d. Accessed March 2019.

[7] Wikipedia. "A journey of a thousand miles begins with a single step." https://en.m.wikipedia.org/wiki/A_journey_of_a_thousand _miles _begins_with_a_single_step. July 7, 2020. Accessed December 17, 2020.